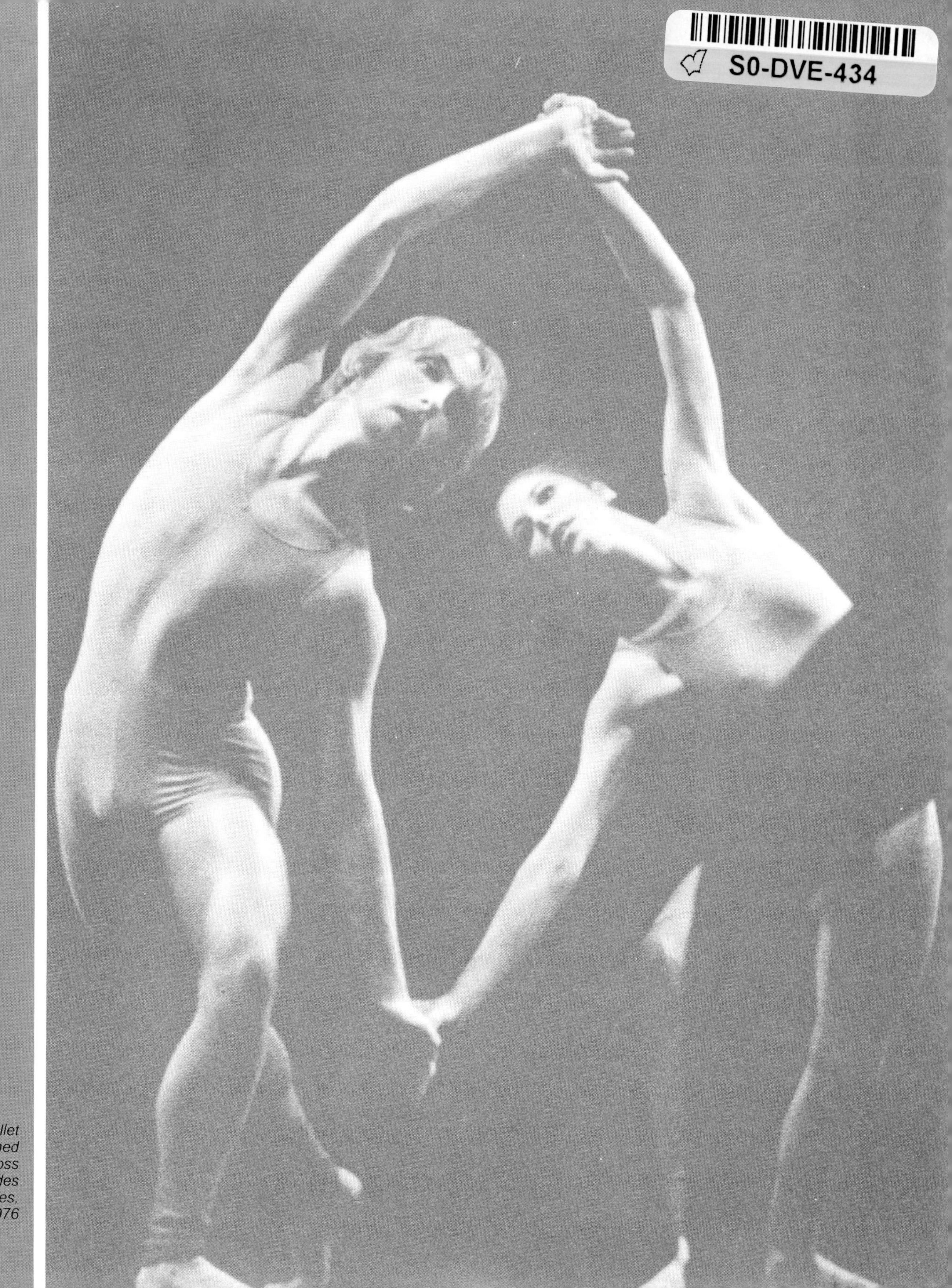

Ballet
choreographed
by Peter Goss
e Théâtre des
amps-Elysées,
Paris, 1976

American Edition published in 1977 by
Barron's Educational Series, Inc.
113 Crossways Park Drive
Woodbury, New York 11797

ISBN 0-8120-5127-0

Printed in France

ODON-JÉRÔME LEMAÎTRE
with the help of Madame YVETTE CHAUVIRÉ
of the Paris Opéra
designed by PHILIPPE LORIN

the dance

COLLECTION
KNOWLEDGE
& TECHNIQUE
youth
a collection supervised by Philippe Lorin

Barron's

Acknowledgements

The author and publisher would like to thank Mr. Rolf Libermann and Mr. Hugh Gall, general director and assistant director of the Paris Opéra, for their help in the preparation of this book. They would particularly like to thank Madame Claude Bessy, directress of the School of Dance, as well as Madame Jacqueline Moreau and Madame Jane Gerodez, teachers, and Madame Nicole Chirpaz of the International Academy of Dance in Paris.

Jacques Kobel and Philippe Lorin would like to thank Anne, Christine, Laurence, Sylvie, Fabrice, Thierry, and all the gymnasts as well as the students of the Paris Opéra School of Dance for their kindness and patience during the photographic sessions. In addition, Philippe Lorin would also like to thank Miss Kahane, librarian at the Opéra, for her very necessary help.

The photographs in this book were taken by Jacques Kobel, with the following exceptions: p. 39, Agence de Press Novotny; p. 41, Francette Levieux; p. 42 on the left, Jack Mitchell; p. 44, Michel Lidrac; pp. 3, 35, 37 and 40, Philippe Lorin.

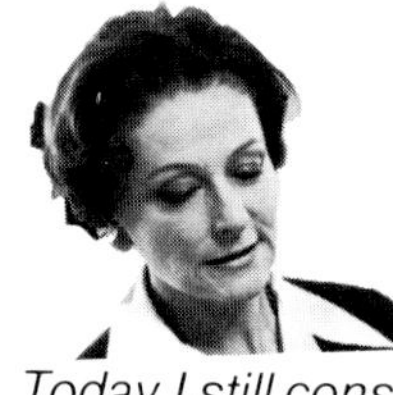

Yvette Chauviré

Today I still consider myself an apprentice in the world of dance because it is a world that is constantly being rediscovered, a voyage that lasts a lifetime.

I guide my students to the path of perfection, training them to overcome the banalities of the every day : to dance is to express the exceptional.

The children who choose to dance enter into an order of beauty, the exploration of a different world.

In these few pages we hope to help them become more aware of their bodies, while discovering those mysterious forces which will compel them to master their art.

Before knowledge and discovery there is nothing but the love for the dance, and the "gift".

In the classical school one is taken up immediately by the hard work and the intense reflection. The dance that we are passing on is a science of the body as well as a symbol of humility : it is also a life of discipline and sacrifice.

Perhaps one day some of you will know this freedom and will achieve this magnificent joy. Even then you will not rest : to dance is to work and to study hard every day, to treat each day as if it were your first.

Above all do not forget that it is music that supports and completes the dancer.

Classical dance is the subtlest of arts, the most physically demanding, the most ethereal and certainly the most beautiful.

Let's discover it together...

From sport to dance

1

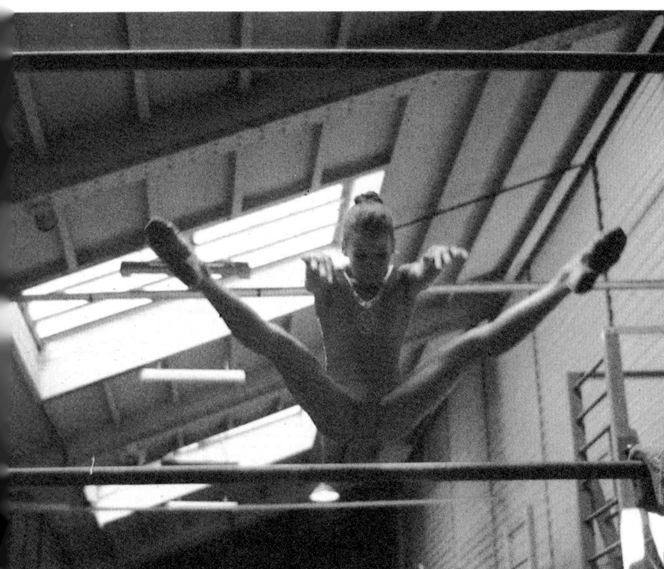

From the strength of an athlete...

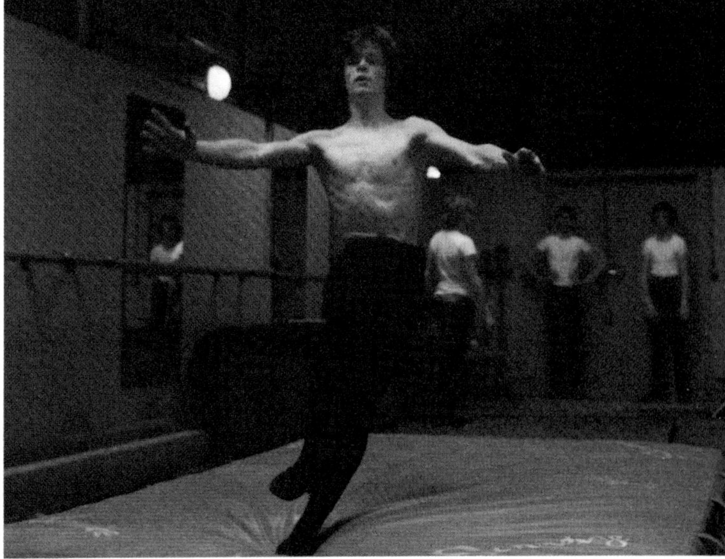

... to the precision of a dancer.

You have surely seen a football match or a rugby game, live or on television. But have your ever seen a ballet?

Do you know that the dance, like sports or any form of recreation, can become a profession, in fact an art: and that it once was the most natural expression of primitive peoples?

Today the machine is replacing man more and more; robots threaten him and he is increasingly troubled by a world forged out of concrete and steel. This is the era of the "industrial society", of man who is too busy taking planes to take a moment for a walk down a country lane, too busy "popping" pills to put his hands to work on the creation of a beautiful object.

In reaction, more and more young people are discovering sports and the dance as means of communicating with the human body. For besides the value found in physical expression there is the deep creative satisfaction they get from performing itself.

If stadiums are jammed, if the crowds are huge at competitive sports, if champions become idols, and if the dance continues to gather a greater following, doubtless it is because each man would like to possess the skill of a rugby or football player, the precision and timing of a boxer, or the ability to dance like the star he is applauding.

Another one of us is at the bar, and on stage at the Palais des Sports in Paris, a virtuoso dances as we ourselves would like to one day. In effect, the great dancers are themselves champions and, as it is true for all other sports and disciplines, their "records" so to speak are constantly being broken.

The gymnast who works with apparatus is, among athletes, the one closest to the dancer. His efforts at limbering, his sense of timing, his aim at balance, particularly while in the air, can all be easily compared to the efforts the dancer makes while at the bar or on the floor.

So in both dancing and athletics man is seen pressing himself into competition with (and against) himself...

Yvette Chauviré's lesson

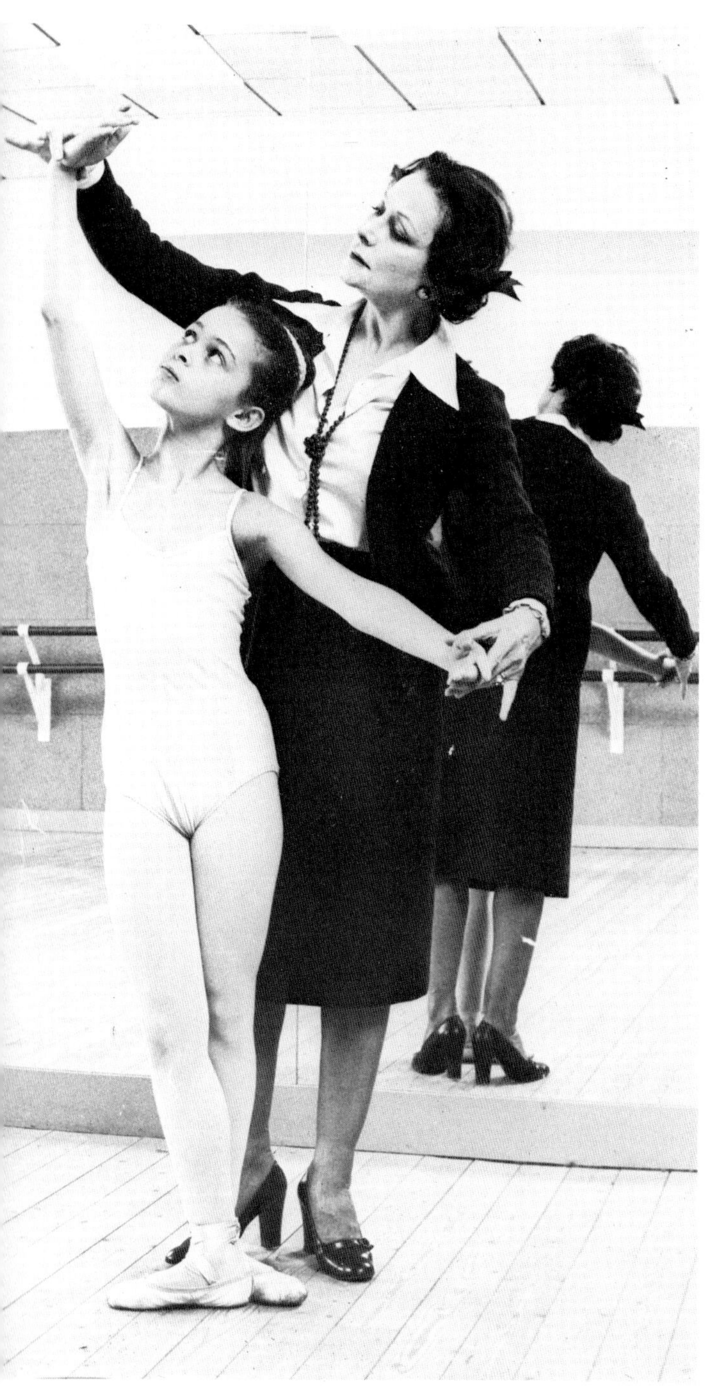

Advice to beginning dancers

For you who are about to discover the dance, it is essential to remember that you move with and are supported by the music.

Learn to look at your teacher, to understand the sense of a well-executed movement. See quickly and well. Your eye and your ear are there to fix the movement into memory. Have a sense of rhythm, a musical ear, and sensitivity.

If the dance is to become your profession - your life - your well-proportioned body will have to be melodious and supple, healthy and well-balanced. Your hands and feet pretty, your head small, your neck long and slender.

You will have to be thin, but not skinny, to have muscles, long legs, fine hands and feet. Finally, you will need to be graceful and to have gracefulness. Never try to copy these qualities in an adult: yours are yours alone.

The greatest gifts are those you yourself bring; little by little you will discover them.

The life of a dancer is simple: in the morning, classes, and in the afternoon, practice; in the evening if you are not performing then you are again at practice. Between these moments, there are the fittings for costumes and meals (not very heavy ones!)

Madame Yvette Chauviré at the Paris Opéra.

2

The studio

For the dancer this is the most important work area. One wall is entirely covered with mirrors, allowing every student to study his work, to verify his efforts, to correct his faults. In a corner, by itself, stands the piano. Very important as all work is done to music.

The bar

Waist high and circling the studio, the bars are fixed to the walls. During training they allow the dancer to maintain his balance with one hand. We call it "at the bar".

Dress

The dress of a dancer consists of stockings going from the ankles to the waist, often in wool in order to encourage transpiration and to help the muscles stay warm. Girls wear a light tunic as well.

The shoes

Traditionally in black leather for boys and pink satin with thick laces that cross around the ankles for girls. When a dancer is working on toe, the toe of the shoe is reinforced.

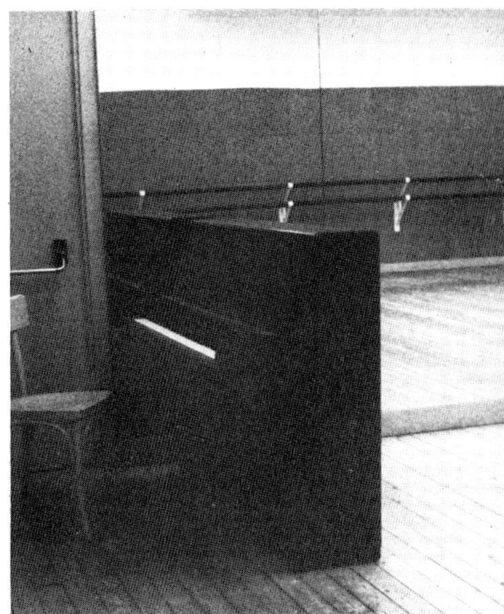

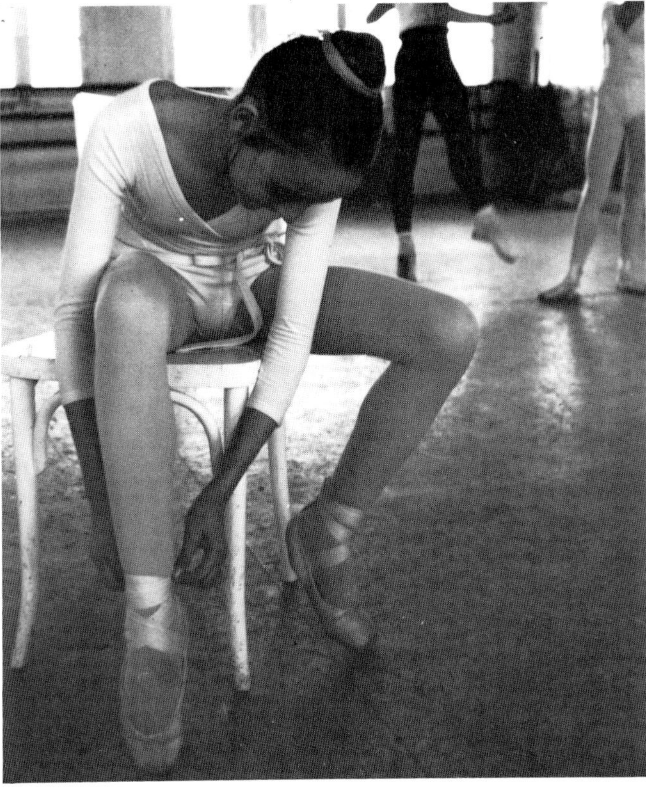

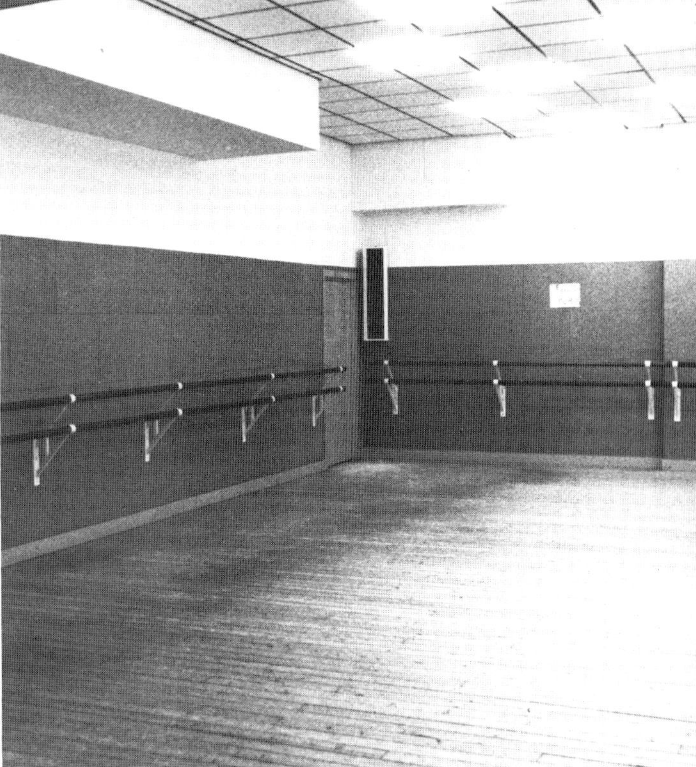

l'en dehors

One of the essential peculiarities of classical dance is what is called "l'en-dehors". It concerns the outward turning of the legs from the base of the trunk, giving the legs a purer line while permitting the dancers to cross the stage from one side to another while still facing the audience.

The legs should appear as much as possible in all the executed movements. The hips should be open, the knee tight and **straight** and the foot, when resting on the ground, resting on three precise points: heel, big toe, and smallest toe. The five positions of classical dance are based on this ABSOLUTE PRINCIPLE and the dancer should try his best to execute it.

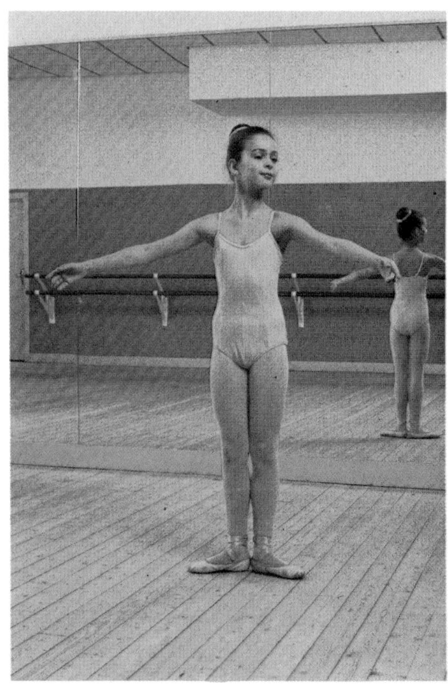

1

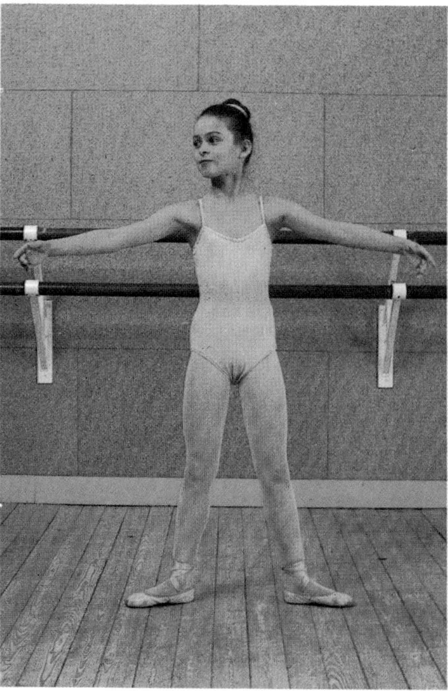

2

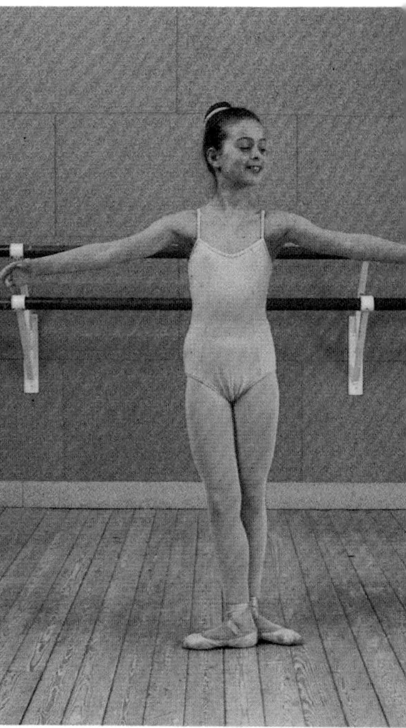

3

the leg positions

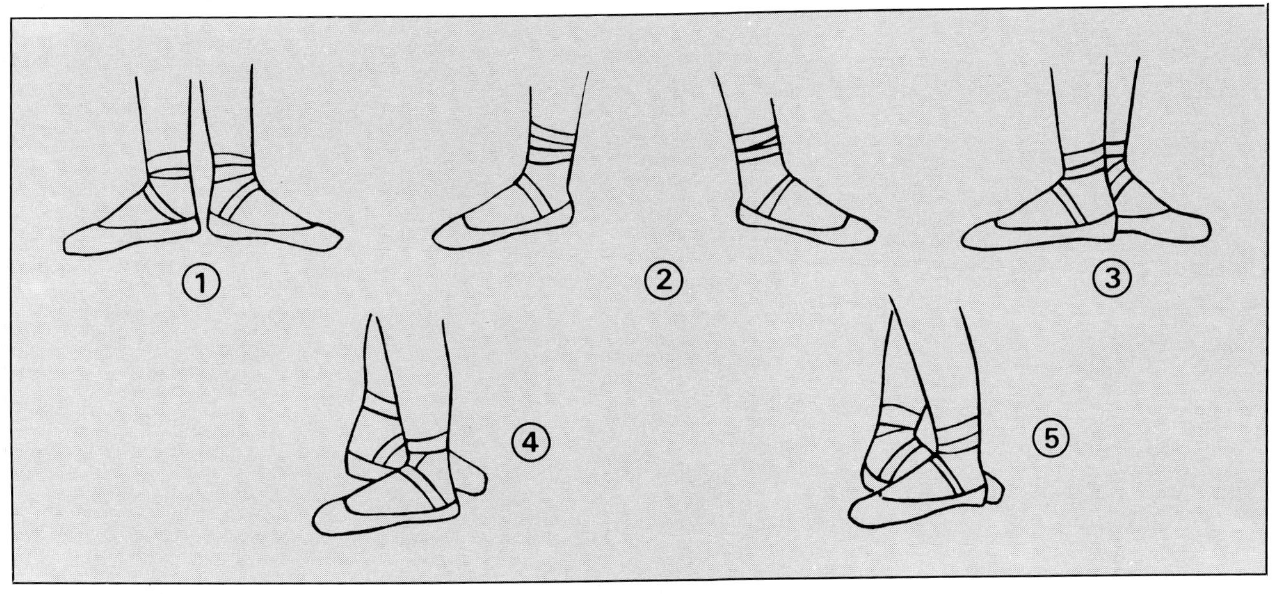

the position of the feet

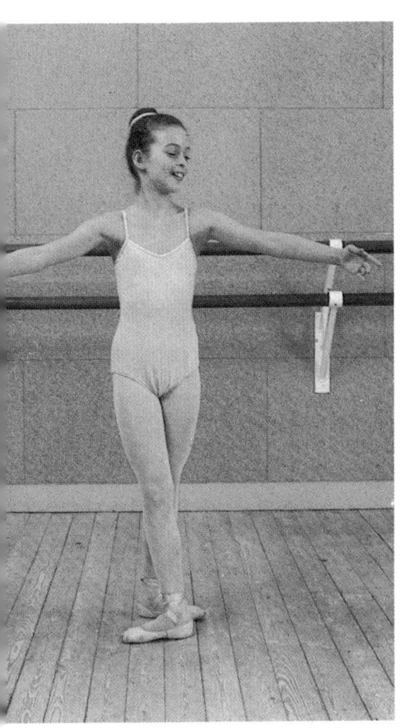

4

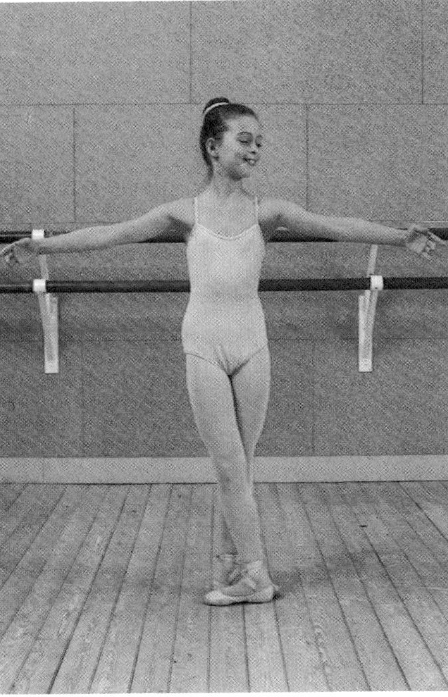

5

1 — In first position, the legs are fully opened out and stretched. The heels touch, the feet form a straight line.

2 — In second position, the same straight line is kept but the legs are separated slightly and the heels do not touch.

3 — In third position the feet are still perfectly facing outwards, the heel of one pressing against the middle of the other.

4 — In fourth position the feet are parallel to one another, still fully opened, with one foot slightly in front of the other.

5 — In fifth position the feet are fully opened and flat against each other, with the toes of one pressing against the heel of the other.

the bar · the floor

The lesson begins at the **bar.**

It concerns a series of exercises that the students execute while standing in profile at, and with one hand being supported by, a bar attached to the wall.

The training continues with a series of "pliés" (bends) in each of the five positions: heels firmly on the floor, raised only at the end of the "plié", legs and feet facing outwards.

What generally follows are the **"dégagés"** (free movements), then the **"ronds de jambes"** (leg movements) either out on the floor or in the air, executed uniquely with the lower portion of the leg in second position, the thigh remaining horizontal and immobile.

Then there are the **"frappés"** and the **"battements",** a series of large and small kicks.

The large "battements" consist of movements wherein the leg is kicked out as high as possible in front of the body, to the side, and in back, with the leg constantly turned out, the supporting leg kept straight and tight.

The small "battements" are full leg and lower leg exercises executed against the floor. Depending on the level of the class the teacher may elaborate on the basic bar exercises by, for example, working on sustained kicks, or balancing on toe.

In general, a series of arm movements called **"grands ports de bras"** (arm and upper body movements) are worked into the lesson, breaking up the concentration on the legs.

Once work at the bar is finished the students take their places out on the **floor** where they execute a series of exercises to develop précision, balance, and beauty: turns, "pirouettes", leaps, and choreographed steps.

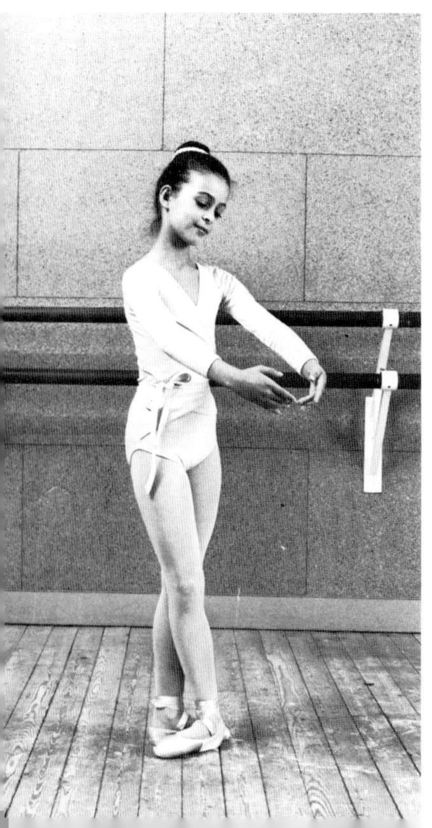

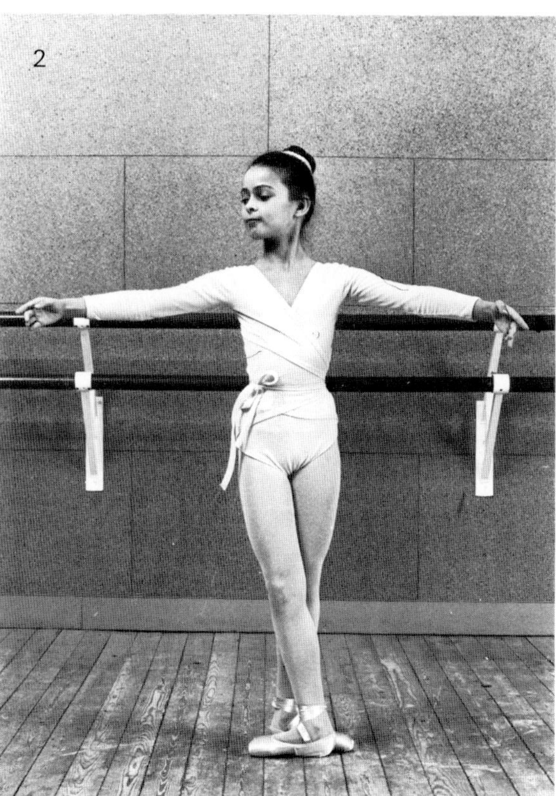

2

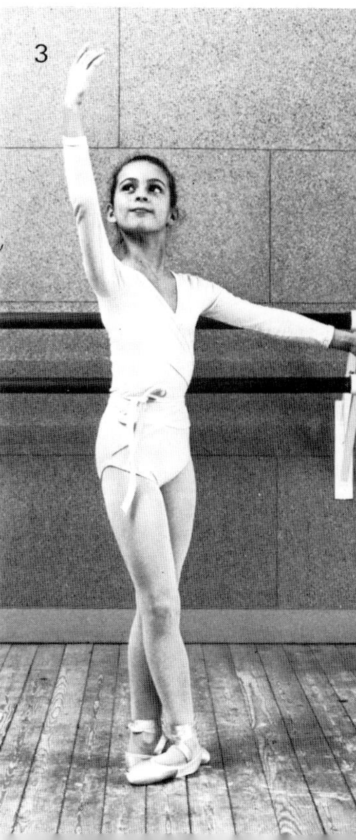

3

the arm positions

2

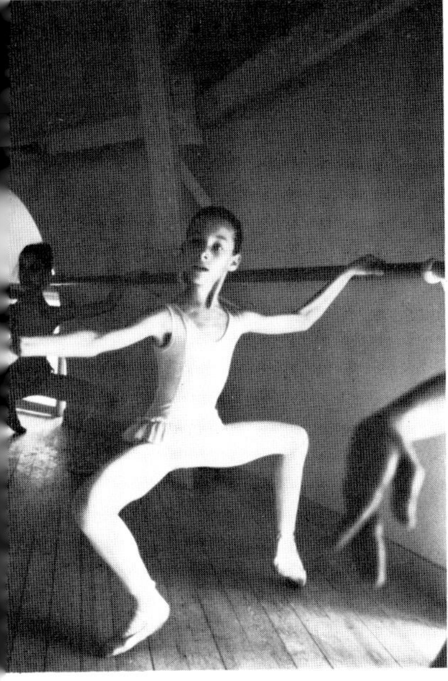

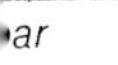

ar

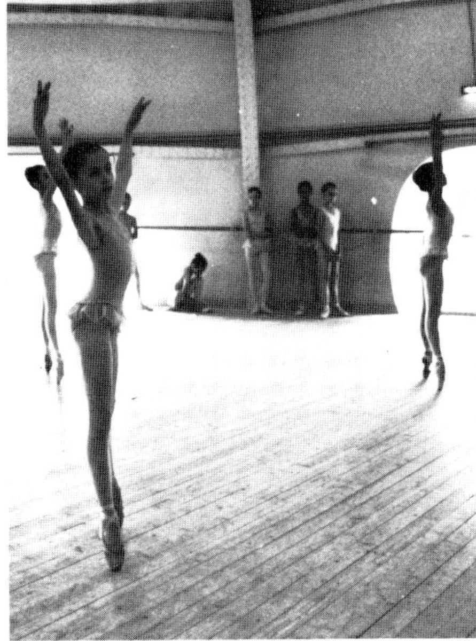

The floor

Five arm positions complement the five leg positions, yet they can be studied independently.

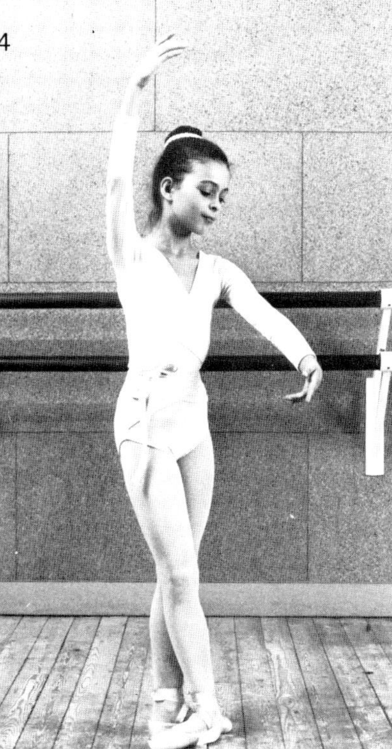

4

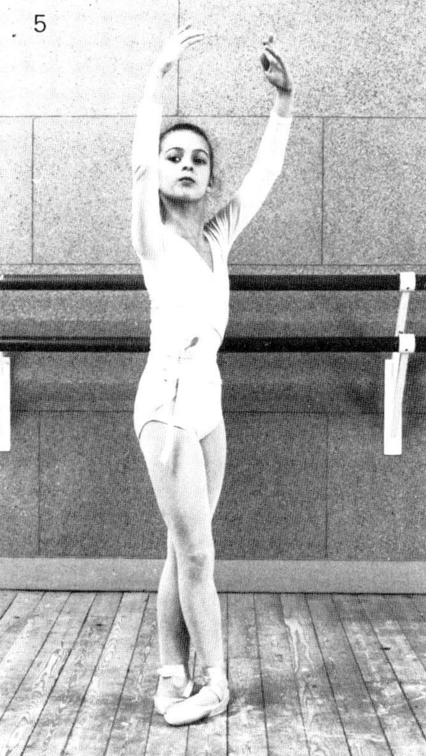

5

1 — Arms symmetrical, held in a circle almost horizontal with the stomach, the palms of the hands turned gently inward.

2 — Arms separated, held lightly to the side in line with the shoulders, elbows rounded, hands in profile.

3 — One arm held out to the side as in the second position, the other in a "demi-couronne" (half-arc) position over the head, the elbow rounded, hands facing inward.

4 — One arm raised above the head as in the third position, the other remaining in second position, palms facing inward.

5 — The two arms form an arc over the head ("en couronne") without hands touching but with them placed slightly in front of the body.

attitude and arabesque · adage

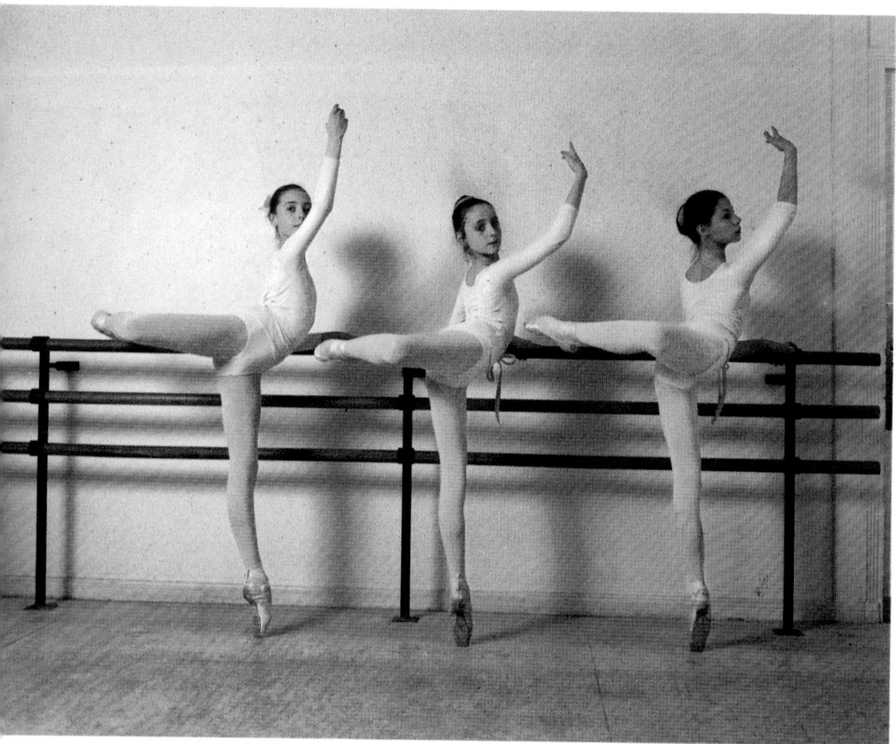

Attitude executed to the side and back

These very beautiful and purely classical positions can be executed face front, in profile, or while turning, as well as with the body open, the legs crossed, on half points, etc...

Attitude

You stand on one straight leg, bend the second, and raise it to form a right angle with the first. The arm corresponding to the raised leg is also raised and slightly rounded while the other arm is held in second position.

Academic arabesque

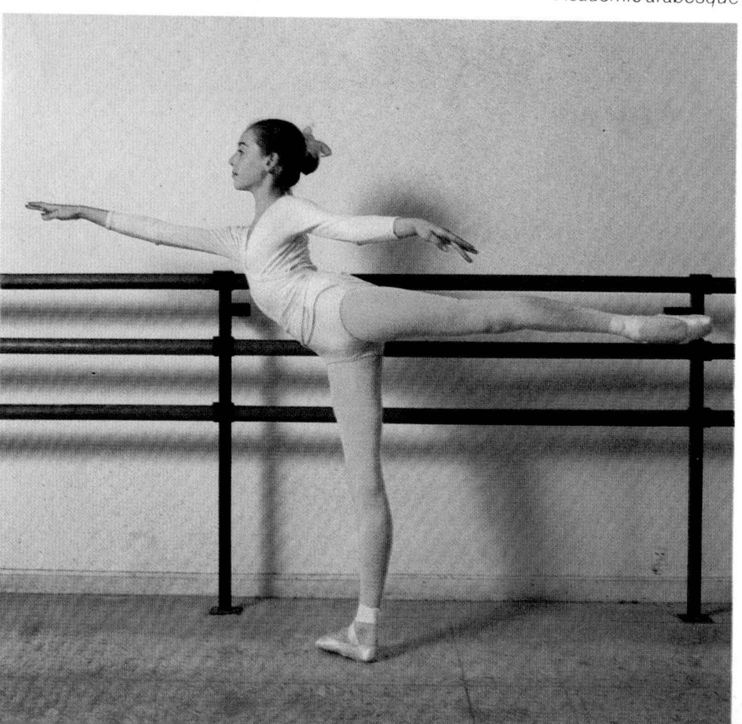

Arabesque

You stand on one leg and extend the other out behind you at a right angle to the first. The arm which is opposite the extended leg is held out straight in front, while the corresponding arm is held back on the side. To succeed at this movement the lower body is well braced and the supporting leg held tight and straight.

2

Adage

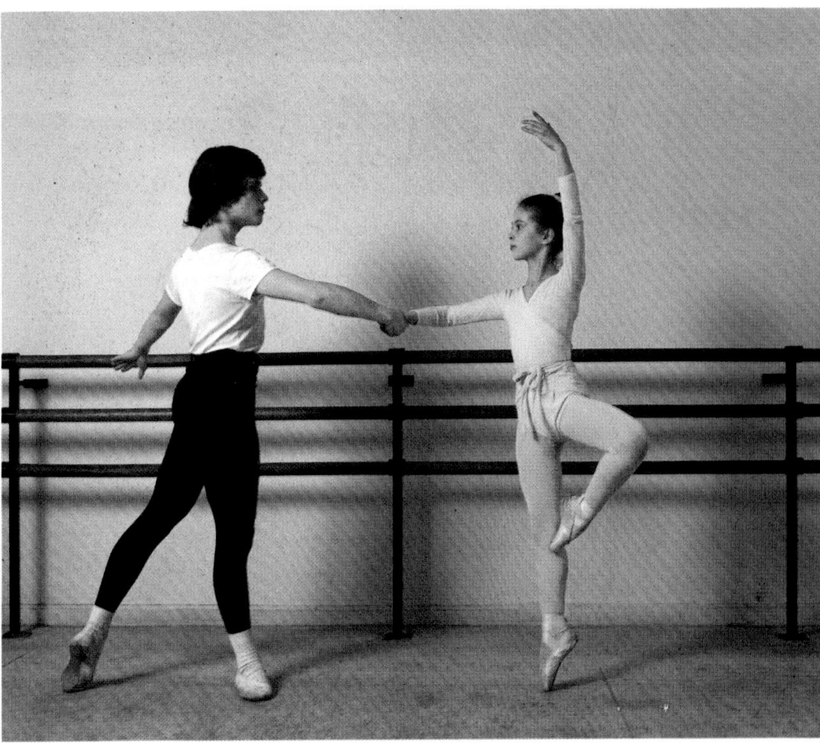

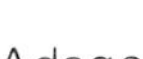

Adage

The "Adage" is an important step in the lesson: students are taught to work out the various combinations offered by the use of the "Attitude" and the "Arabesque" positions.
The "Adage" is, besides an expression of sensitivity, a preparation for a "pas de deux", a love duet danced by a dancer and her partner.

Romantic, or interpretive Arabesque

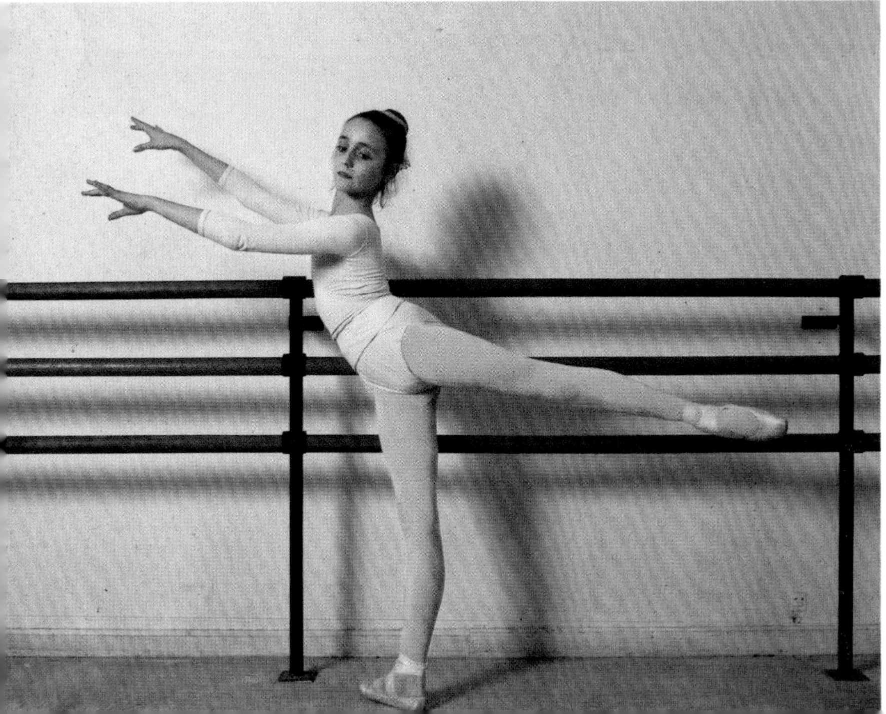

pas de bourrée

The " Pas de Bourrée " consists of three steps executed with the body completely open and facing front. The first of these steps is executed with the foot placed flat on the floor, the following two on half toe or full toe. At times, the " Pas de Bourrée " precedes a pause.

Starting in fifth position, right foot in front.

Do a demi-plié (half-bend), bending the left leg in back or the right. Bring the left leg to the floor on half toe (demi-pointe) and shift your weight to this leg. The axis of the body is to the right.

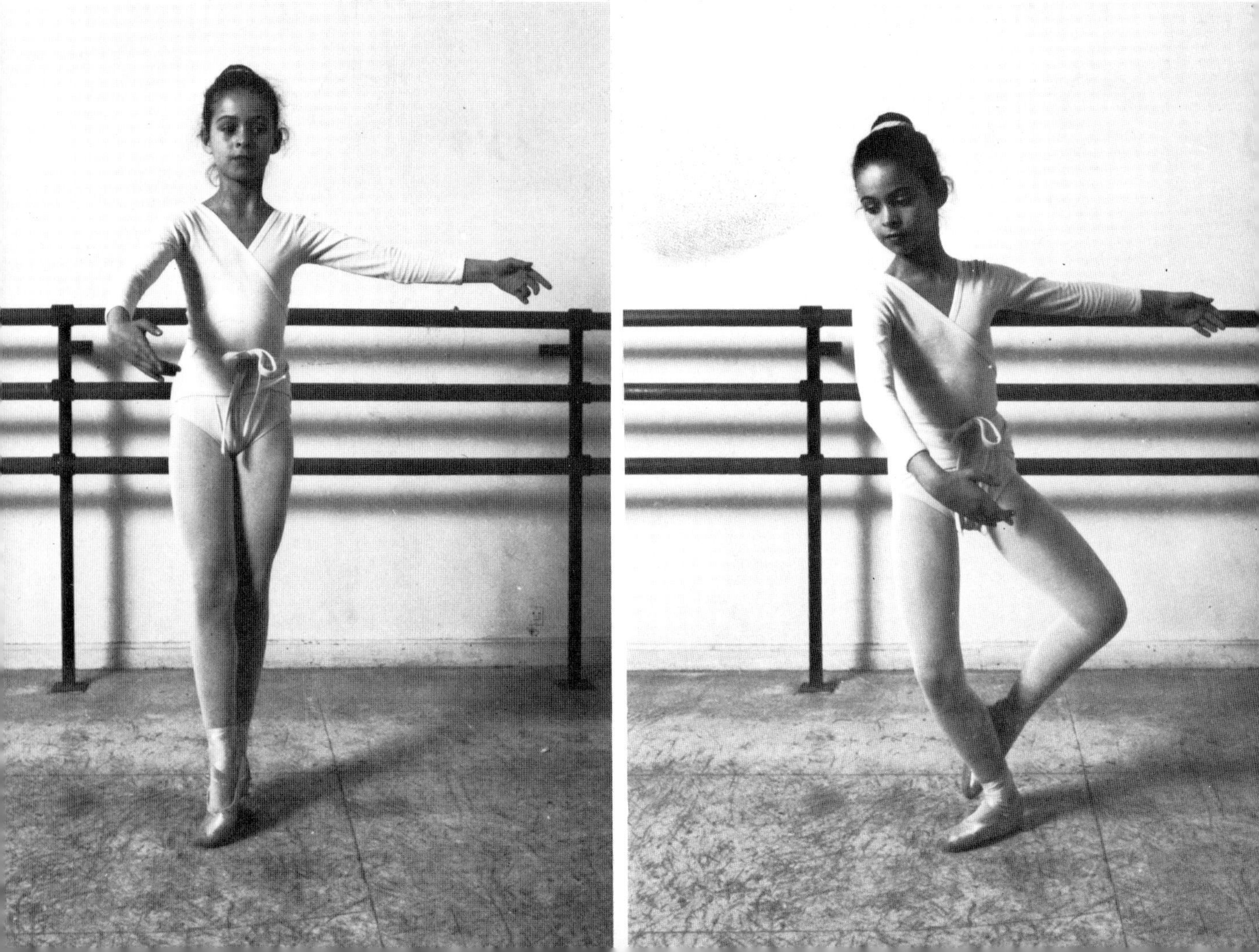

Attention!

The body must remain straight. Notice that you have changed your foot position during this exercise.

Stretch out both legs and continue on to the second position on half toe.

Finally bring the left leg in front of you in the fifth position, again in demi-plié, after having subtley changed the axis of the body by leading with the left shoulder.

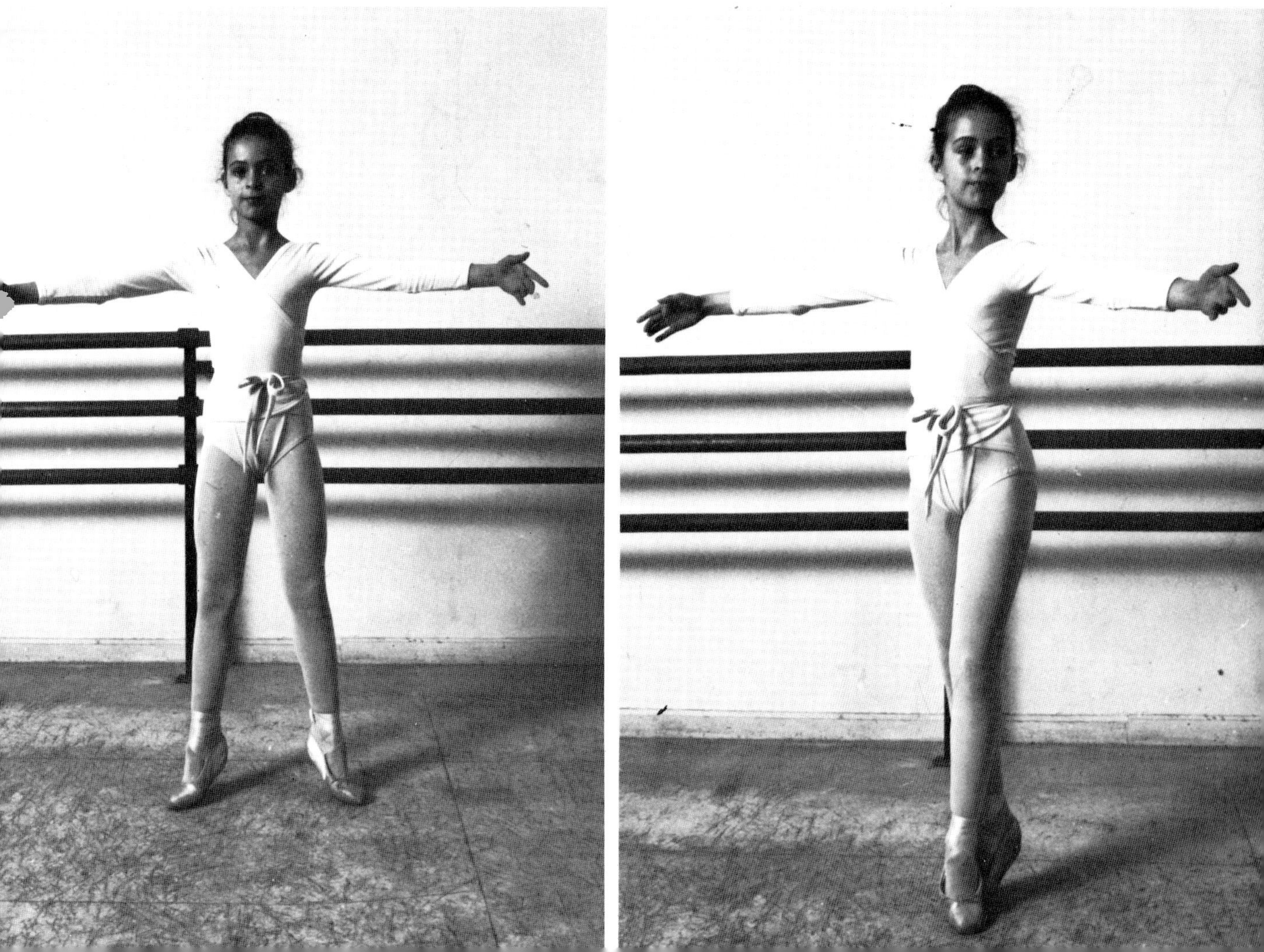

pas de basque

Pas de Basque

The "Pas de Basque" is composed of sliding movements. It is executed by sweeping one leg in a circle around the body, meeting the second leg, freeing this leg to move forward and ending by the first leg joining the second leg in fifth position.

Make a demi-plié in fifth position. The right foot is stretched to a point and is fully extended in front of the body. Pass through the fourth position, compose a half circle while passing through second position with the point of the right foot. Arriving at a demi-plié in first position, shift the body weight while bringing the leg around the right side. Place the left leg in front, finish by joining the legs in fifth position.

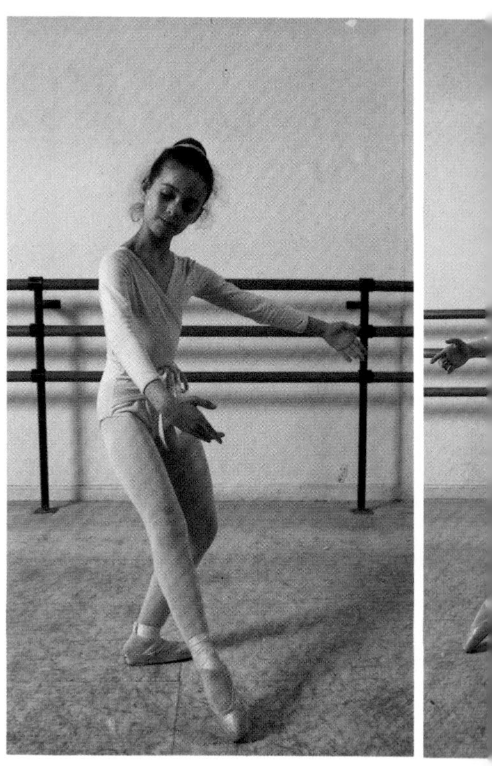

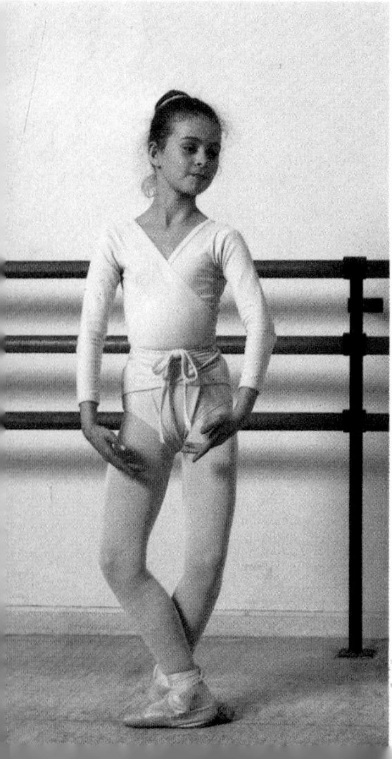

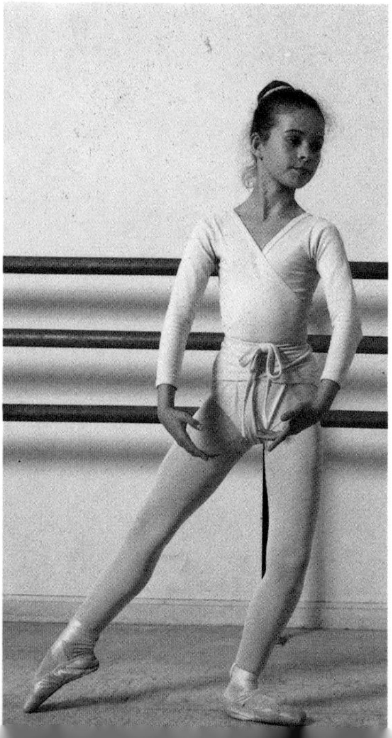

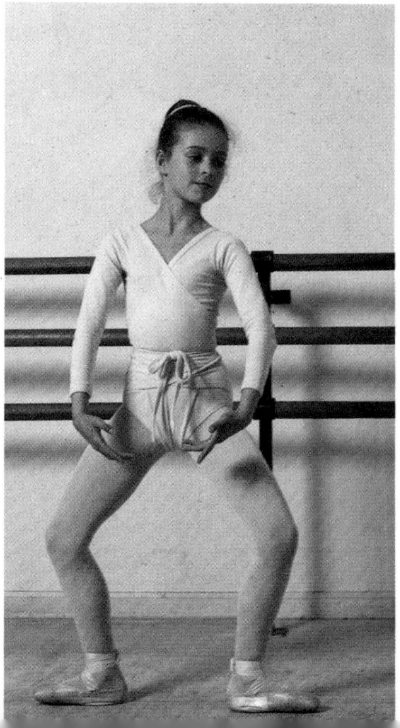

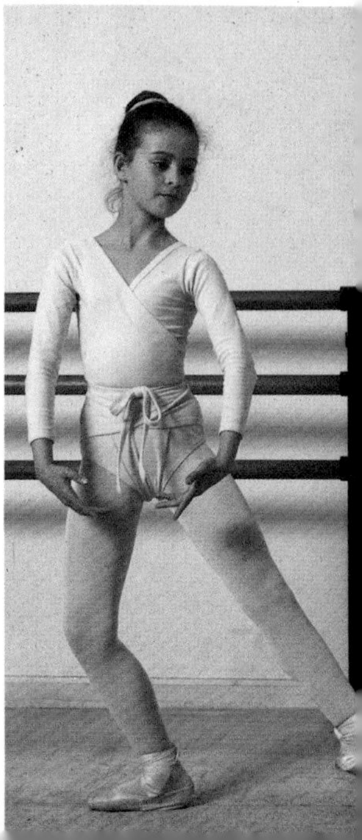

glissade

2

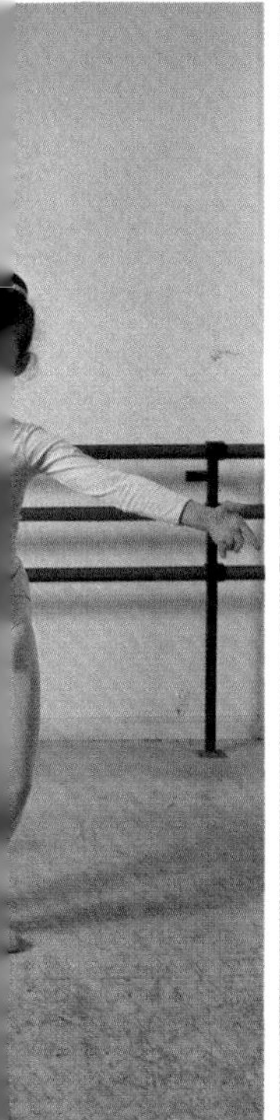
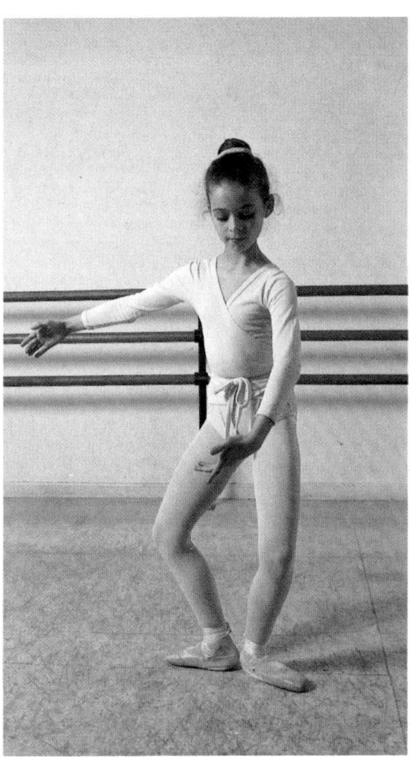
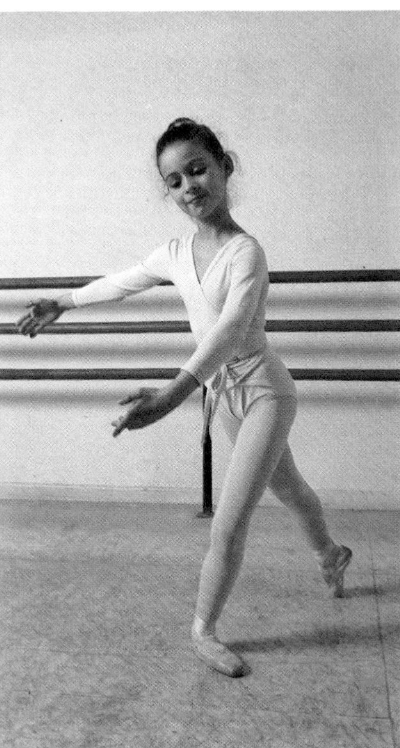
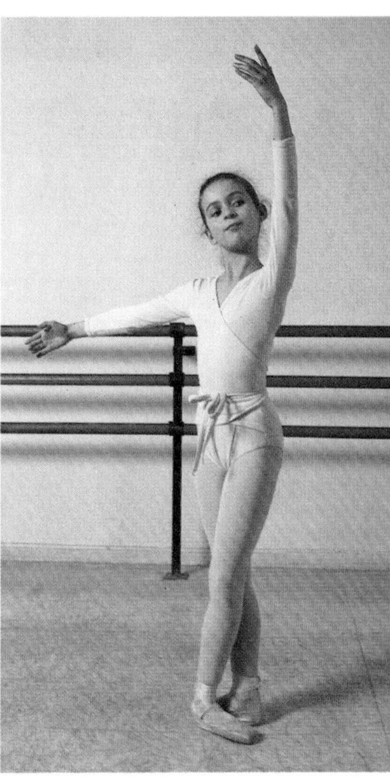
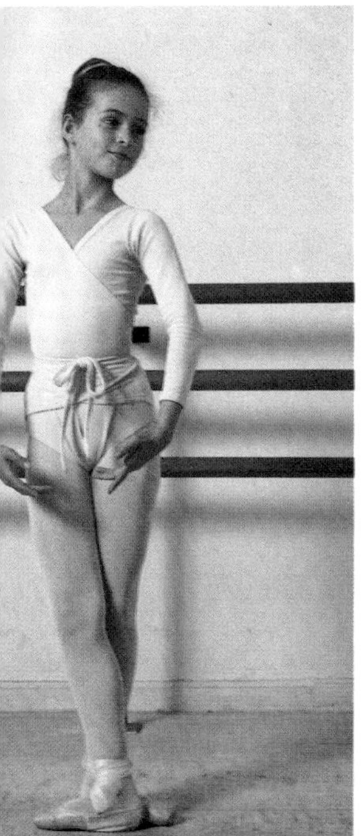

Glissade.

The "Glissade" is a small movement on the ground, often used as preparation for other movements and leaps. It is executed with or without changing the feet.

Make a demi-plié in fifth position, left foot behind the right, and point the right leg to the side. Lightly balance your weight on the right leg, and quickly pass through the second position. Bend the right leg slightly, straighten the right leg and finish in fifth position.

leap · changing of the feet

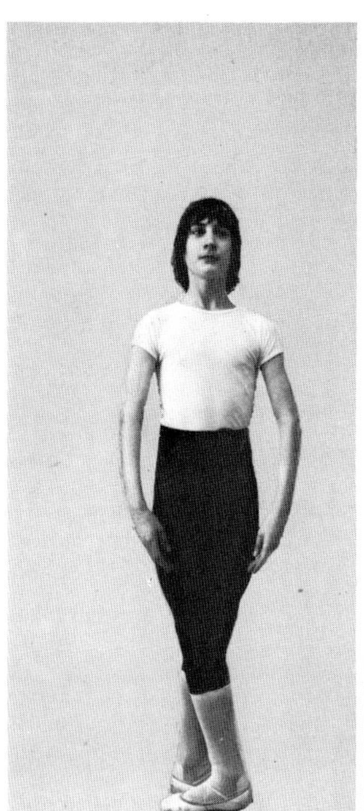
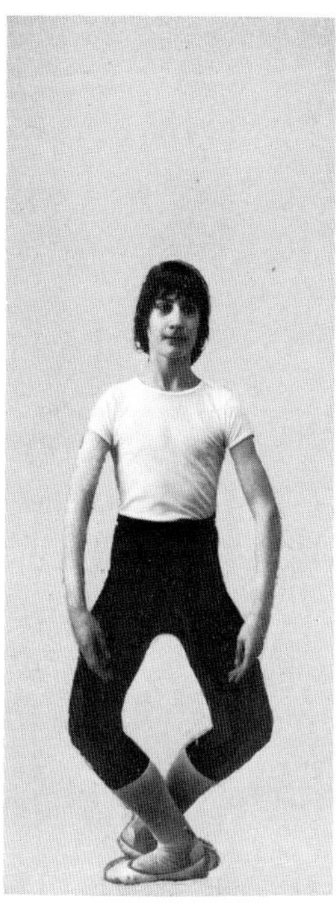
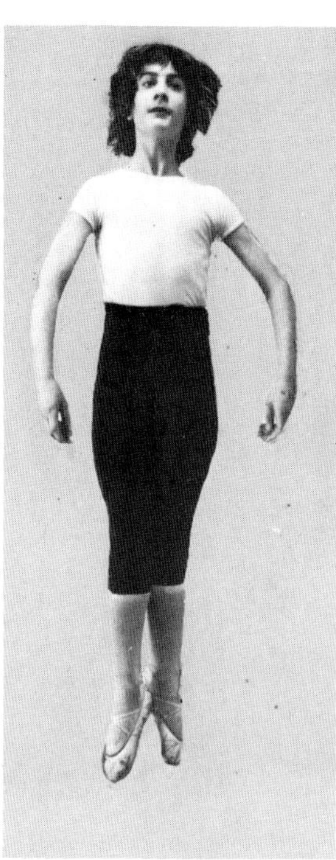
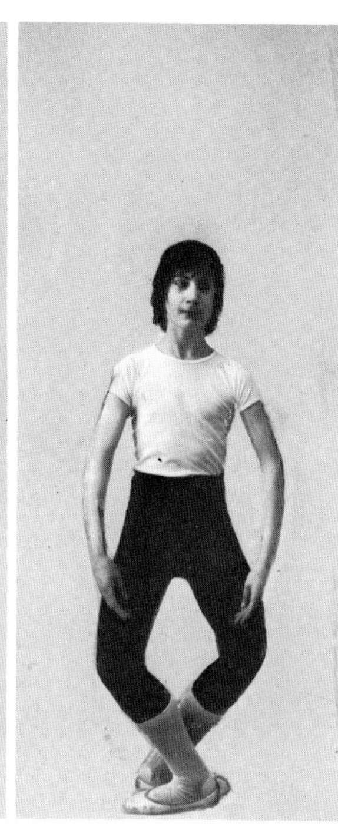
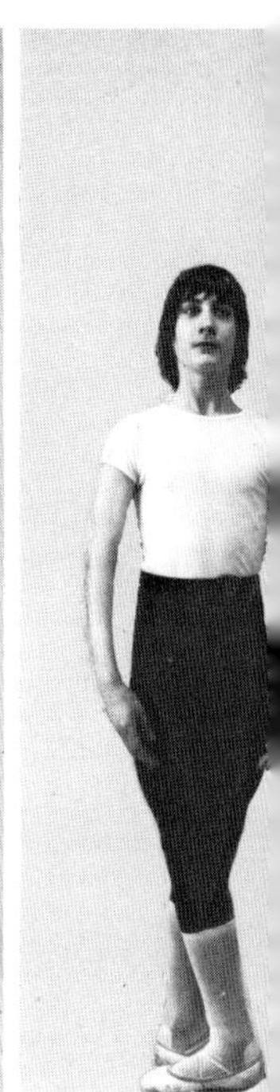

Changing of the feet

Changing of the feet can end in an "Entrechat III". The right foot is in front of the left before leaving the floor. Upon completion of the leap, the left foot is in front.

It consists of a vertical jump from the fifth position, prepared by a demi-plié.

Once in the air the legs are opened in first position with the feet stretched to a full point. Before touching ground again the feet are reversed and at the completion of the jump the legs are in fifth position.

During this leap, as with all other leaps, the head should be lifted high "off" the shoulders. Ther arms should appear to be totally relaxed. The changing of the feet should take place just before touching the ground.

2

Soubresaut

The "Soubresaut" corresponds in principle to the "Entrechat I". It is a simple vertical leap executed in place in which the feet remain close together, one in front of the other, toes pointed.

Staying in fith position, in demi-plié, you jump in place while stretching the legs and knees and pointing the feet. Then you finish in fifth position, after a demi-plié.

When the leap is finished the body is slightly arched forward so that is still appears to be floating.

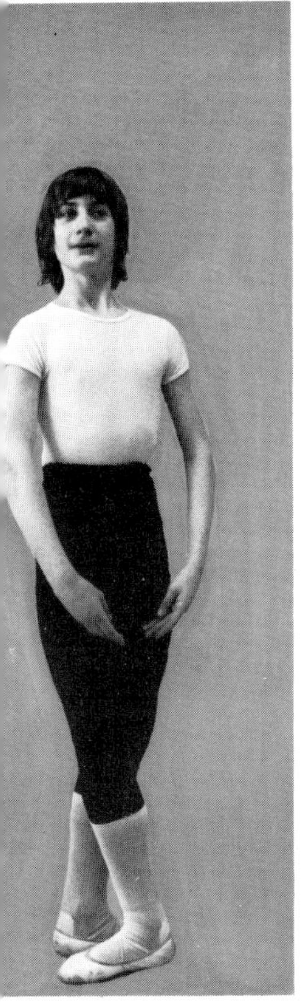
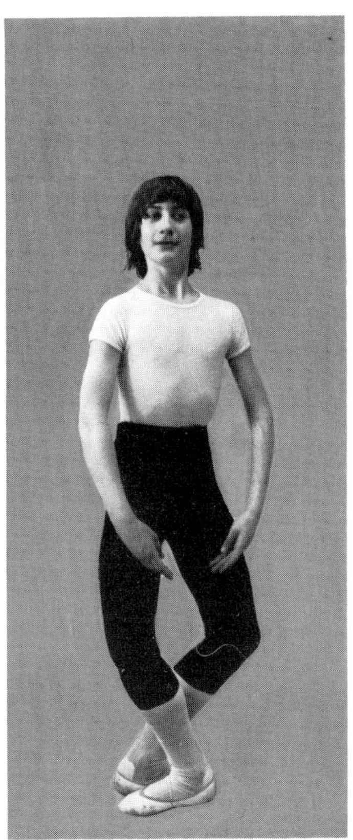
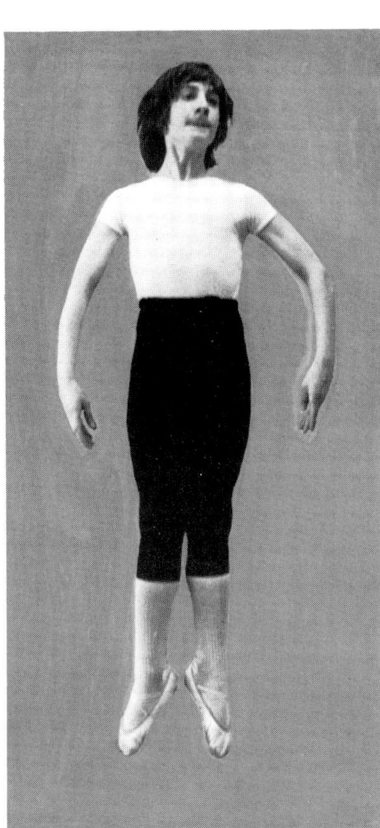
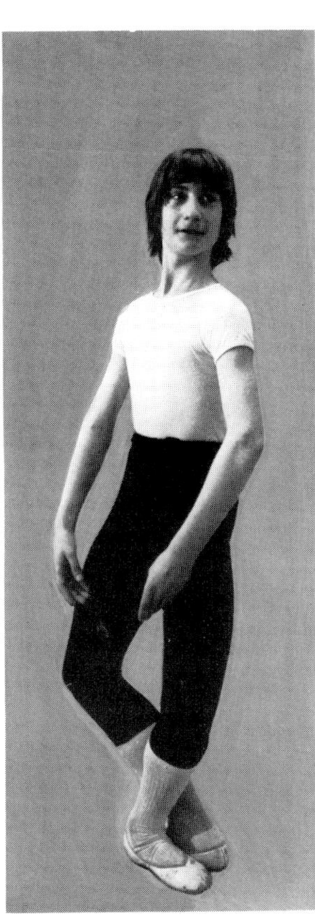

entrechat · assemblés

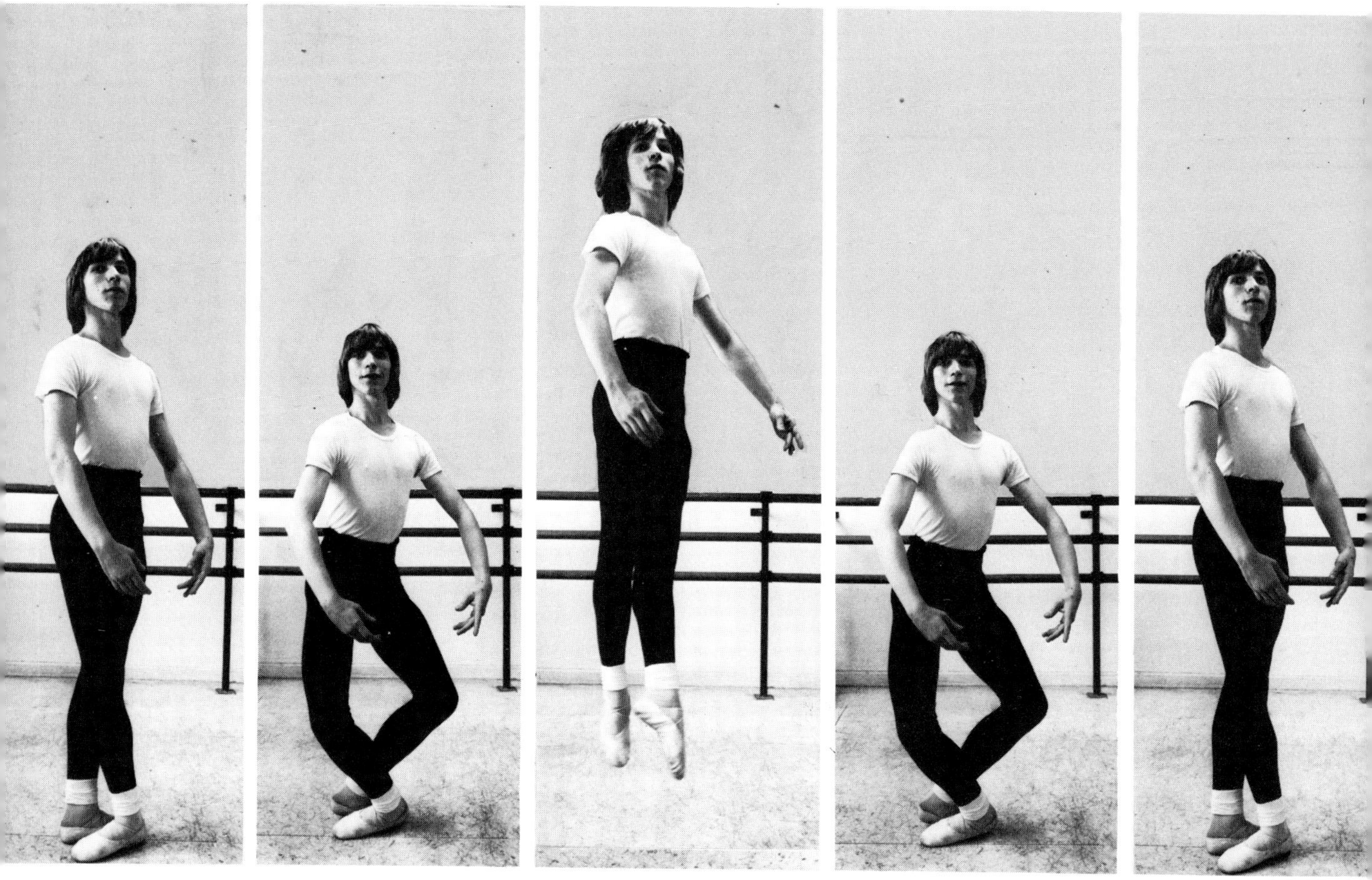

So that an "Assemblé" is beautifully executed, the legs must come together and touch just before landing on the floor.

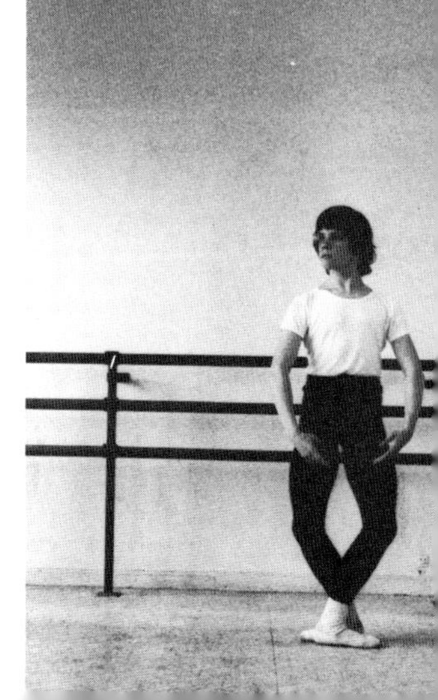

Entrechat

The " Entrechat " like the " Soubresaut ", is, generally speaking, a vertical leap during which the legs cross before landing.

Entrechat I : equivalent to a " soubresaut ".
Entrechat II : equivalent to a changing of the feet.
Entrechat III : equivalent to a changing of the feet plus a " petit battement " (slight kick or thrust) executed by the front leg.
Entrechat IV : the front leg passes behind and then returns to the front before landing.
Entrechat V : same as above, after the execution of a kick by the forward foot.
Entrechat VI : a necessary figure: leap, kick to the back, in place, in front, then land in fifth position.

You jump while quickly crossing the front leg behind and returning it to the front in fifth position.

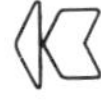

It is essential that the " Entrechat " be accomplished at the height of the calves and not at that of the feet; if it is low, it gives an impression of utter and unsightly confusion.

Assemblés

An " Assemblé " is simply a joining of the legs while off the ground.

You are in fifth position, in demi-plié, the left foot forward. As you leap the two legs meet in the air. You land in your original position, but with the right foot in front.

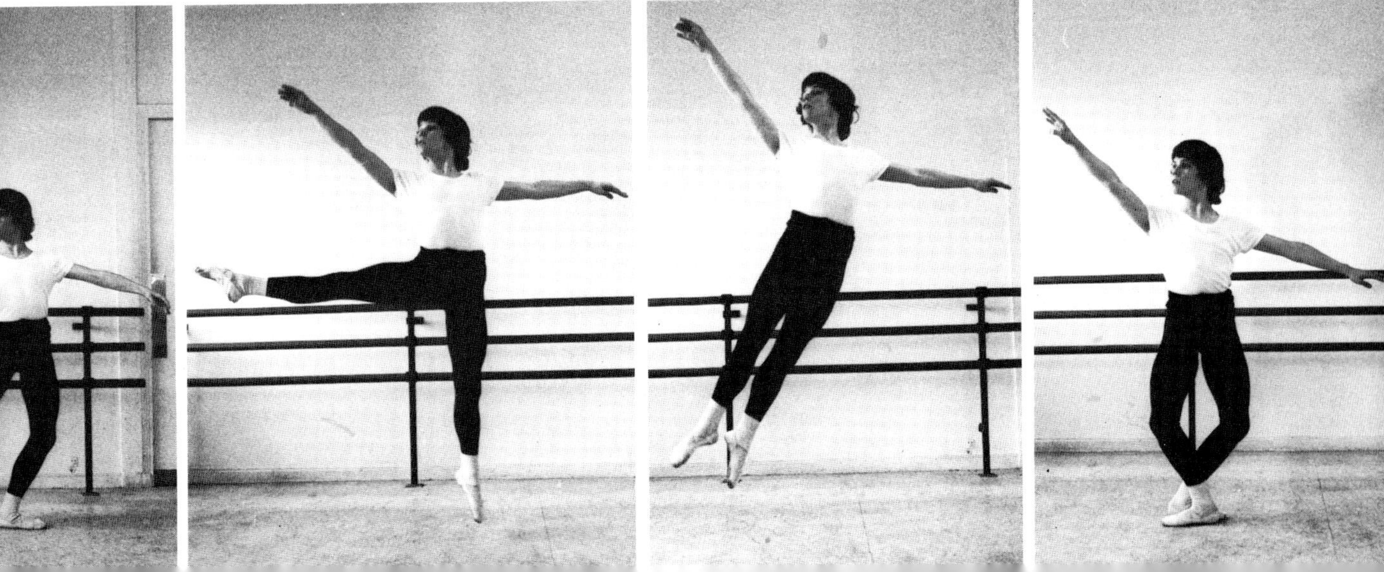

échappés · jetés

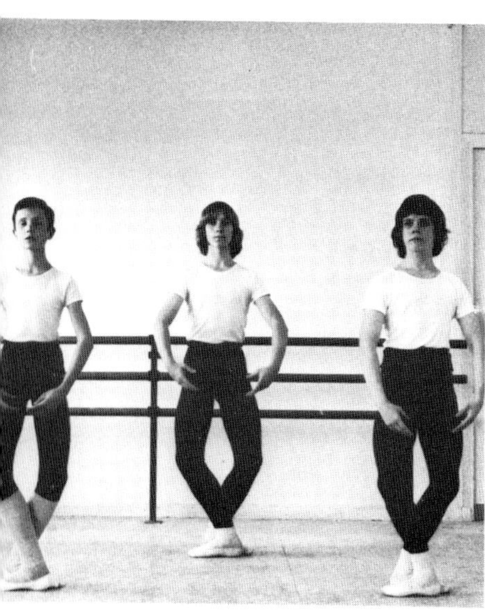

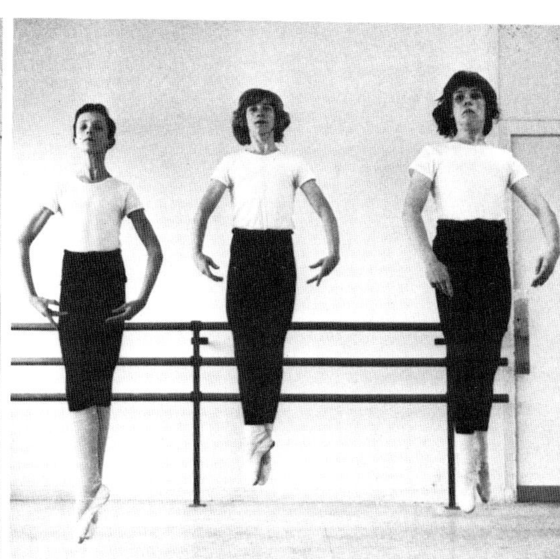

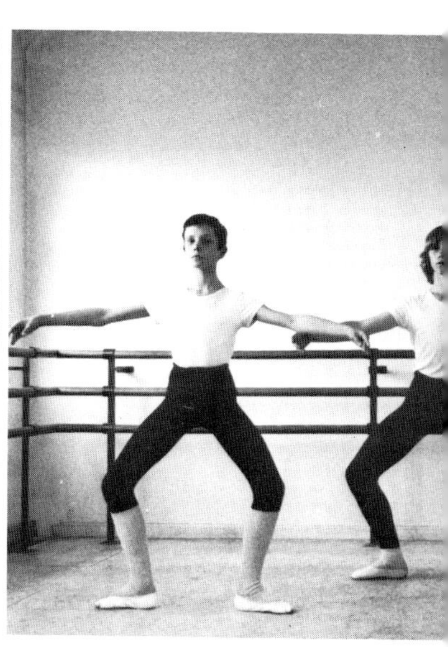

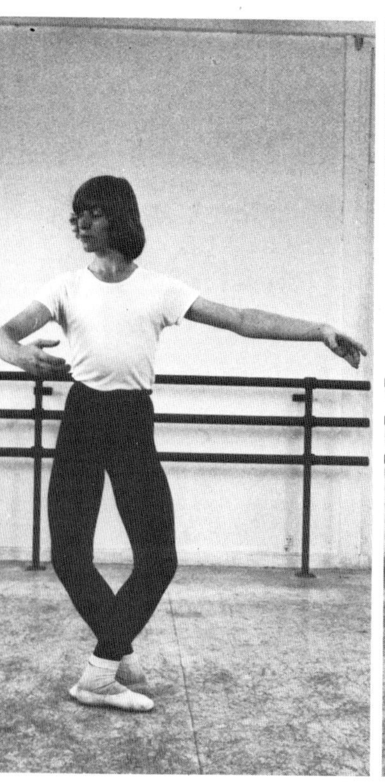

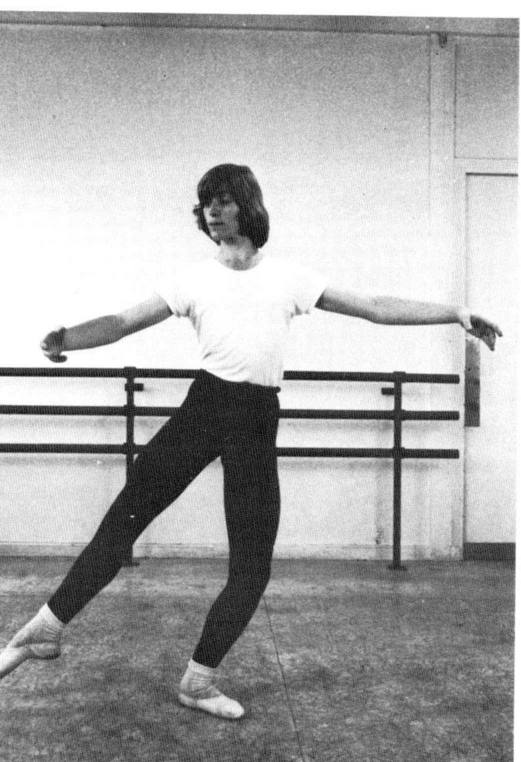

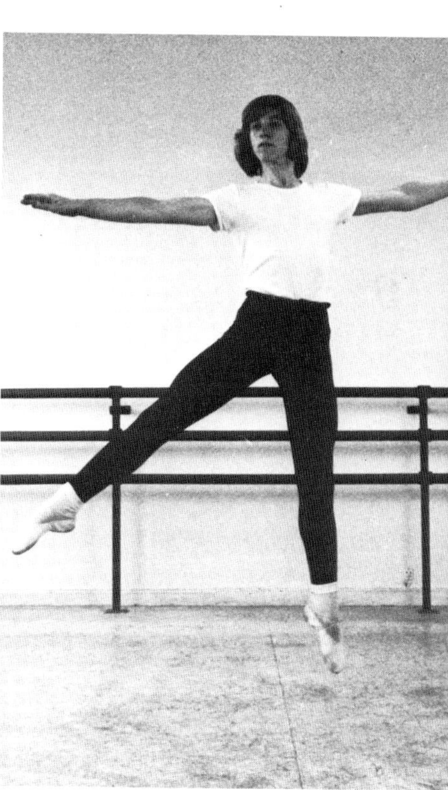

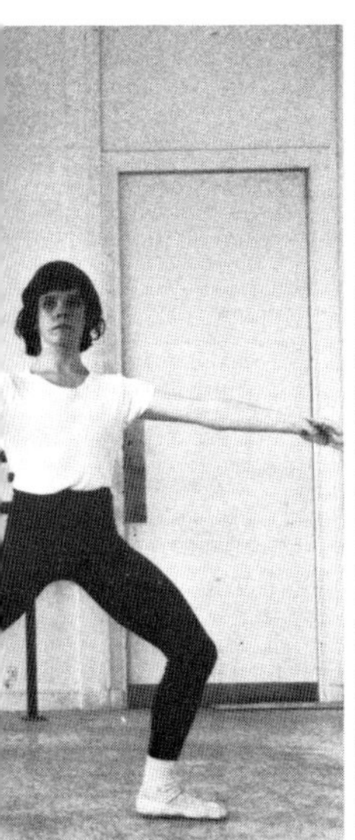

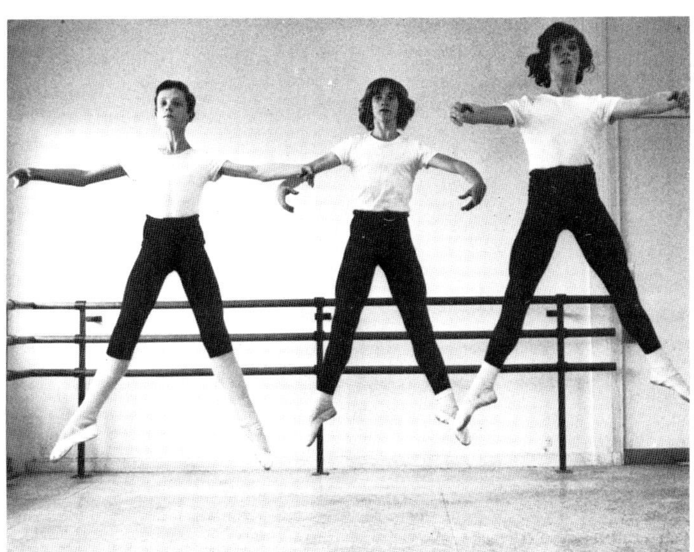

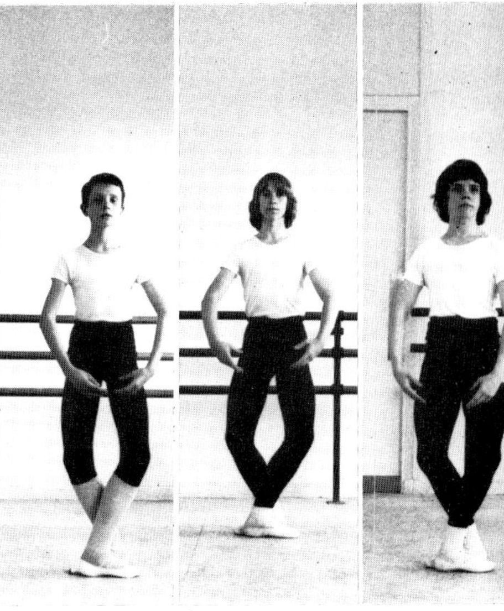

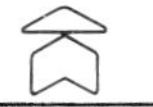

Echappés

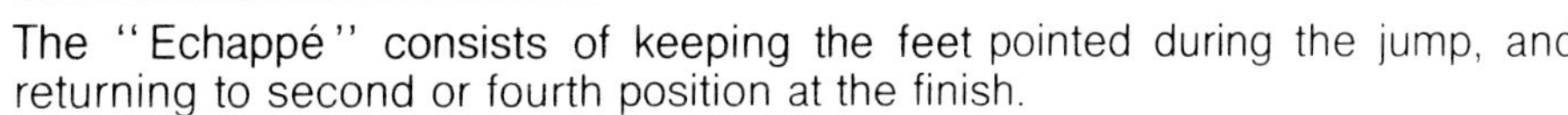

The "Echappé" consists of keeping the feet pointed during the jump, and returning to second or fourth position at the finish.

Beginning in fifth position, right foot forward, you jump, keeping your feet together. Pass on to second position while in the air, legs extended.
You land in second position, in plié. You immediately jump again, into second position, and land in fifth position, the left foot forward.

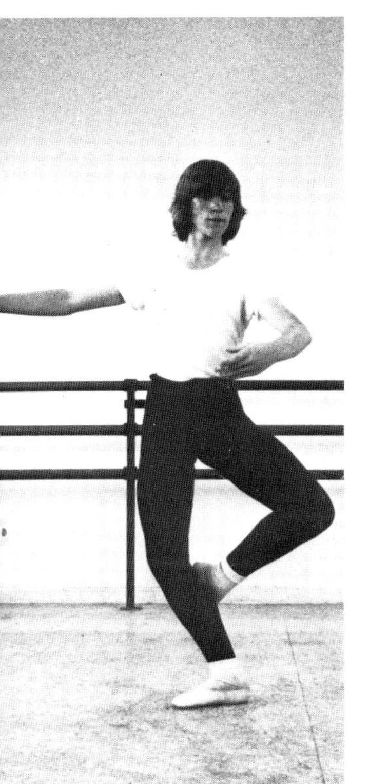

> *The body should not fall forward during the plié. Be sure your weight is equally distributed over the whole foot before leaping.*
>
> *"Jetés" can be accomplished in any direction. They are either "Petits" (small) or "Grands" (large). A dancer can cover a great distance with the "Grands Jetés".*

Jetés

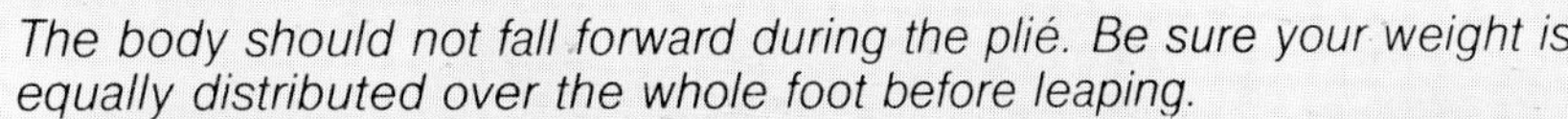

A "Jeté" is a leap from one leg to the other. Often it is accompanied by a "Glissade". However, it can also simply be a series of jumps from one foot to the other.
For example, at first the right leg comes from behind the left and is extended while the left leg supports the body for the lift. Upon landing it is the right leg which is now supporting the body, the left which is extended, and so on.
You bend the legs in fifth position, right foot in back : then you throw the right leg into second position in the air.
You lean on the bent left leg, push off into the air and bring the right leg in front of the left for the landing, and so on.

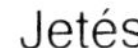

sissone · cabriole

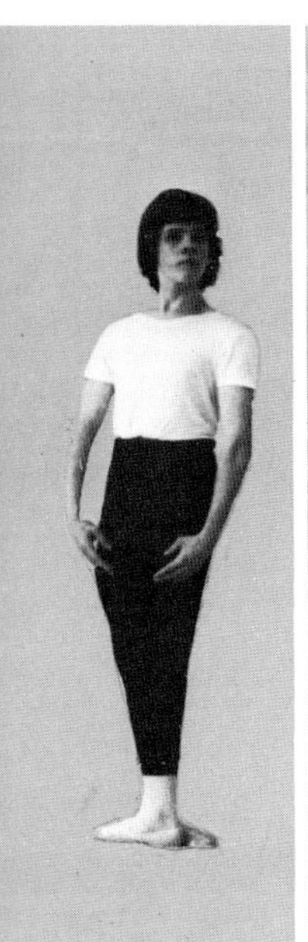
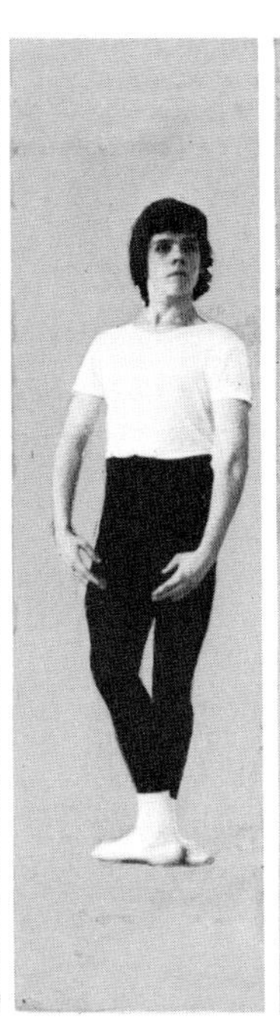
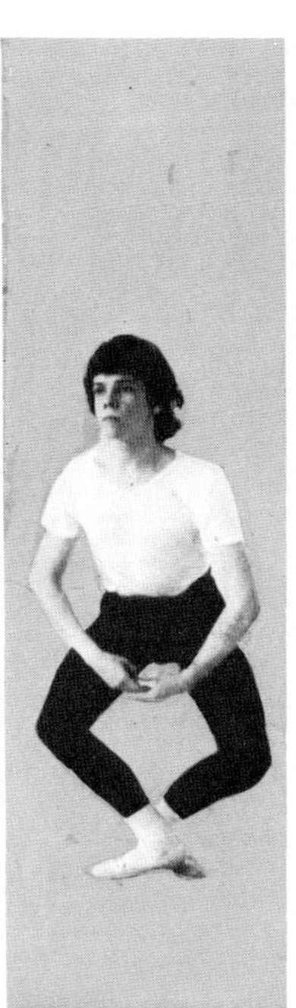
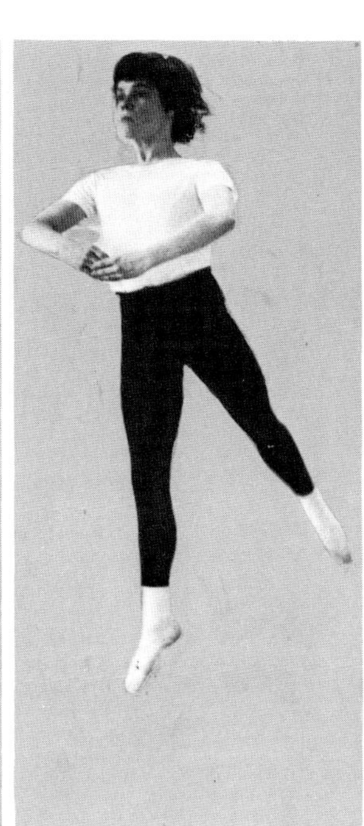
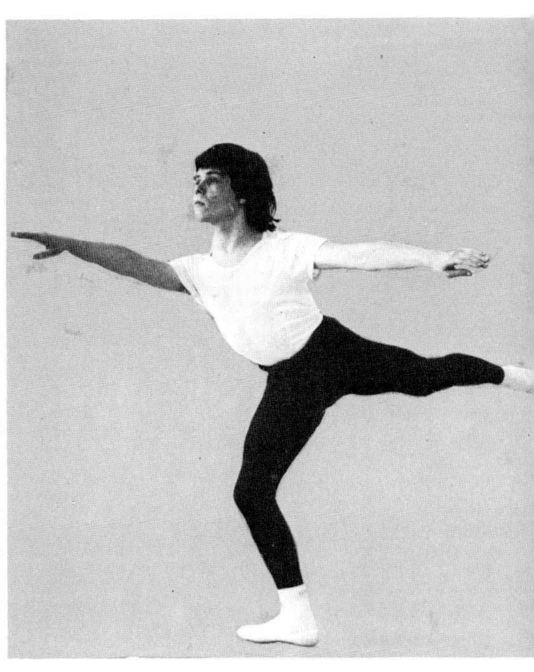

Cabriole

During this leap the dancer releases one leg, and both legs come together at the finish. If the leap is not clean, the supporting leg will be hit at the calf. You are in fifth position, in demi-plié, left foot forward. Release the right leg into second position. Leap on the left leg while maintaining the right leg in the air. Land in fifth position, in demi-plié, right foot forward.

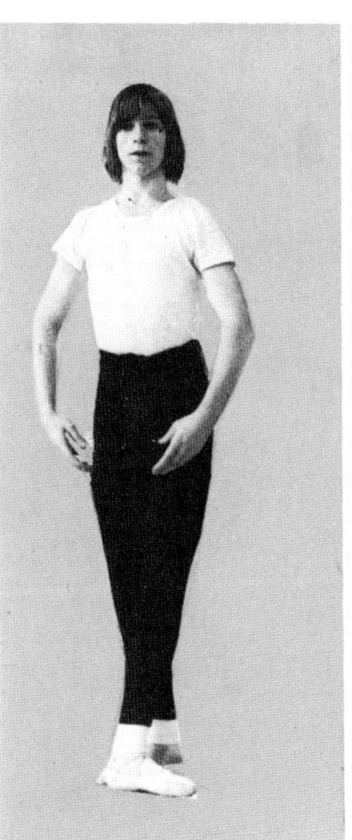
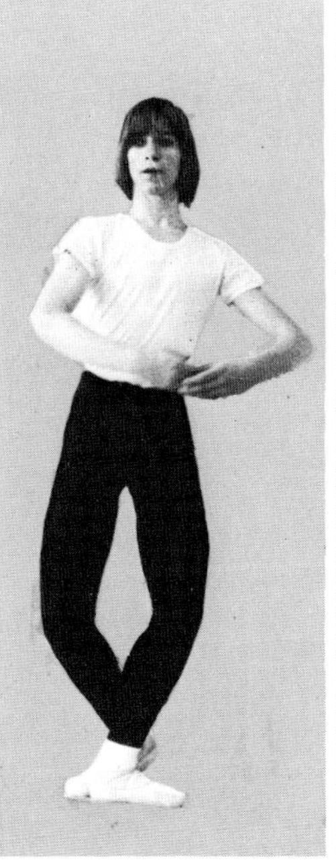
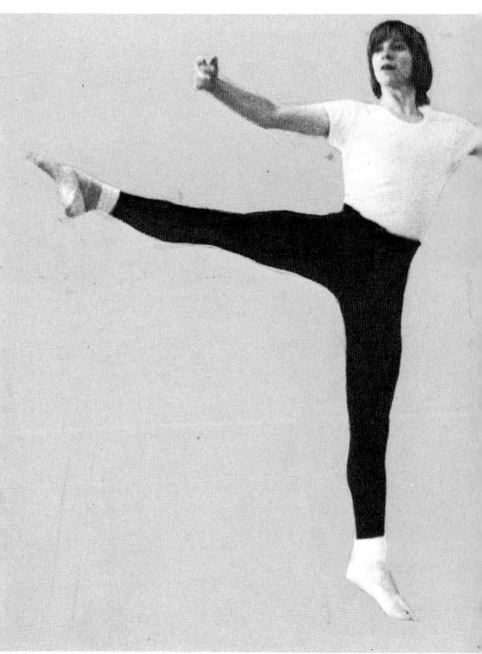

2

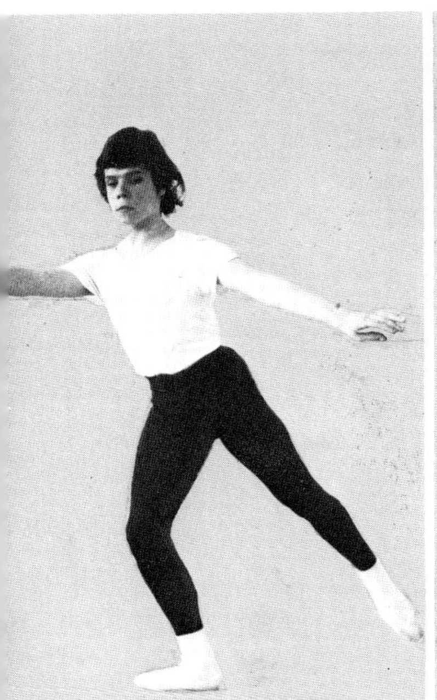

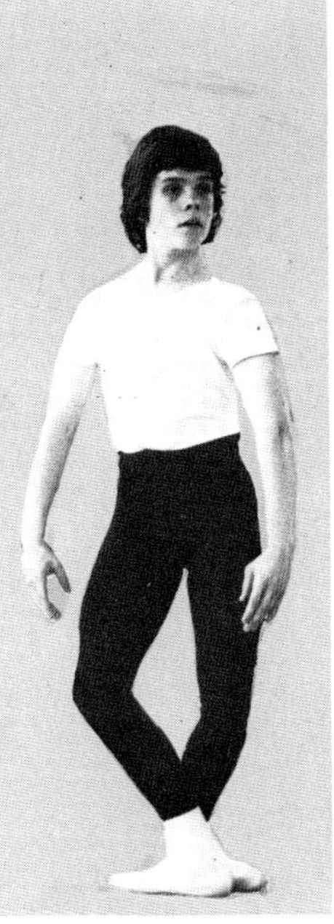

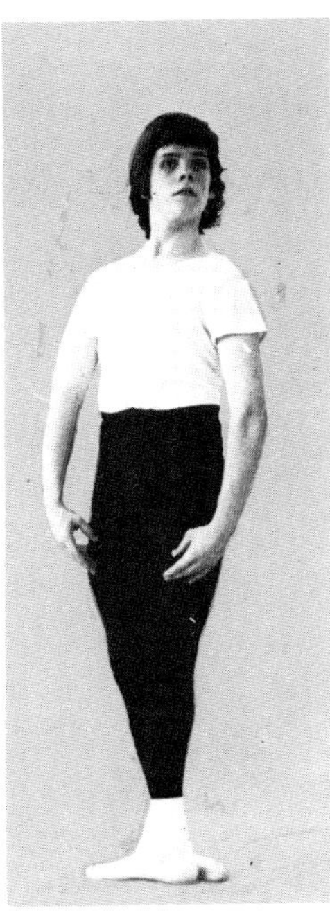

Sissone

Both legs are used to thrust the body into the air, one leg supports it upon landing. The dancer gains ground during the leap.

Plié in fifth position, right foot forward.

Then jump on the right foot, at the same time opening the left leg while in the air into second position. Finish in fifth position, in demi-plié, right foot forward. This movement can be accomplished forwards or backwards, to the right or left.

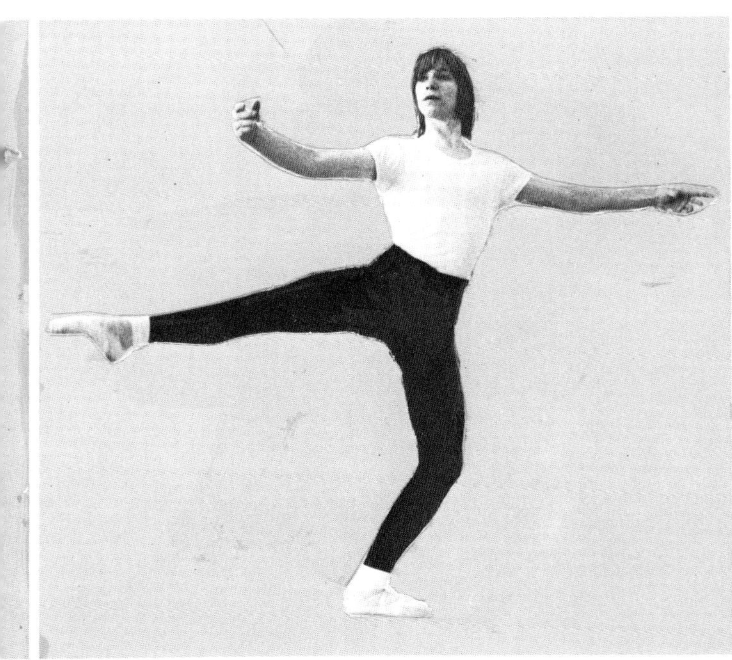

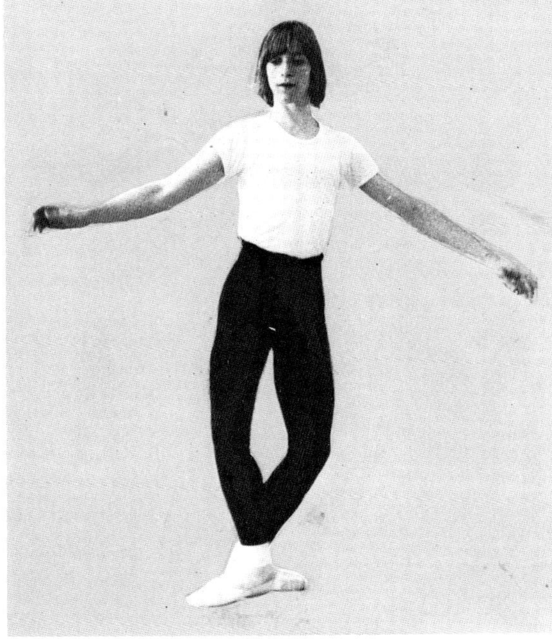

pirouettes · turning in the air

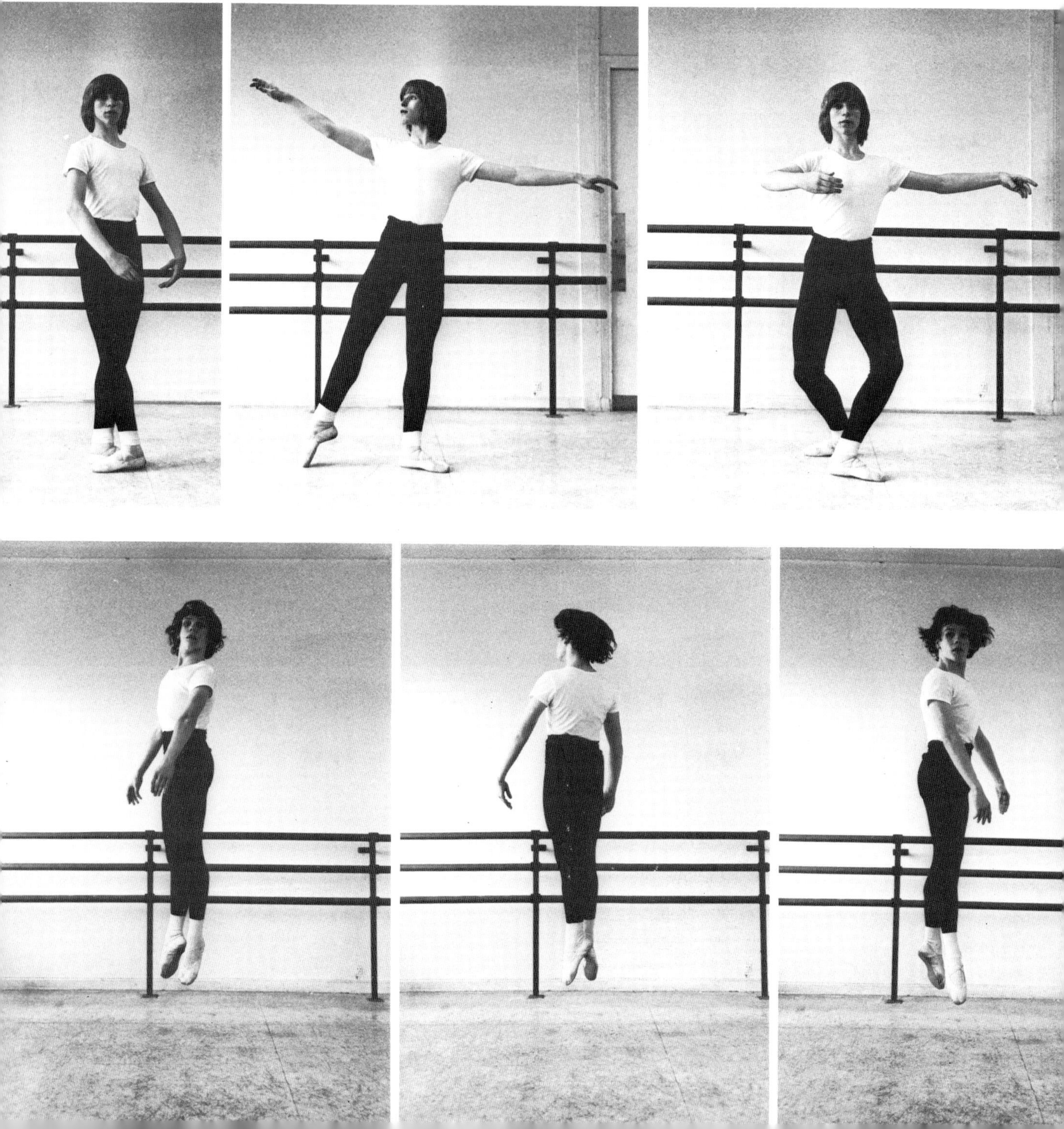

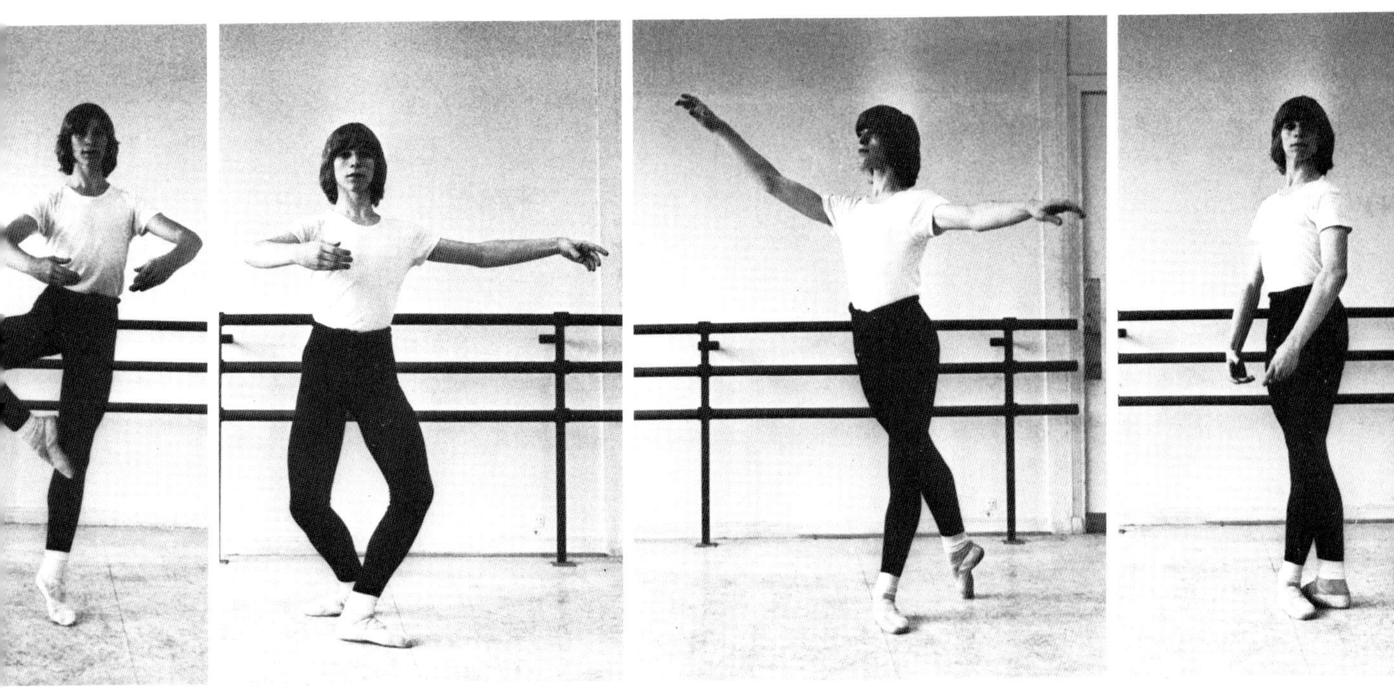

Pirouettes

Movement executed in one spot, during which the dancer turns while keeping his weight on one foot, always on half-toe for the boys, often full toe for the girls.
These turns are done with the body turned out, turned in, the arms held close, quickly, or while in "attitude" or "arabesque".
Other turns are executed while the dancer is moving, whether on one foot, or two as in the "déboulés" (unwindings).

> *To keep a fixed axis while turning, the dancer has to tighten the lower part of the body, sense a straight line beginning at the neck and ending at the lower back, and realize that the way he uses his head will help him keep his balance. His head must move quicker than his body so that during the turn he is facing the public as often as possible. Pirouettes must be done in quick succession, without hesitation.*
>
> *It is always preferable to land in the same spot after executing a turn in the air. Make sure that the knees are straight, and the toes pointed low.*

Turning in the air

This movement is executed during a leap and only by men. Beginning in the fifth position the dancer turns up to three times in the air before landing in either fifth position or on the knees.

The Paris Opéra

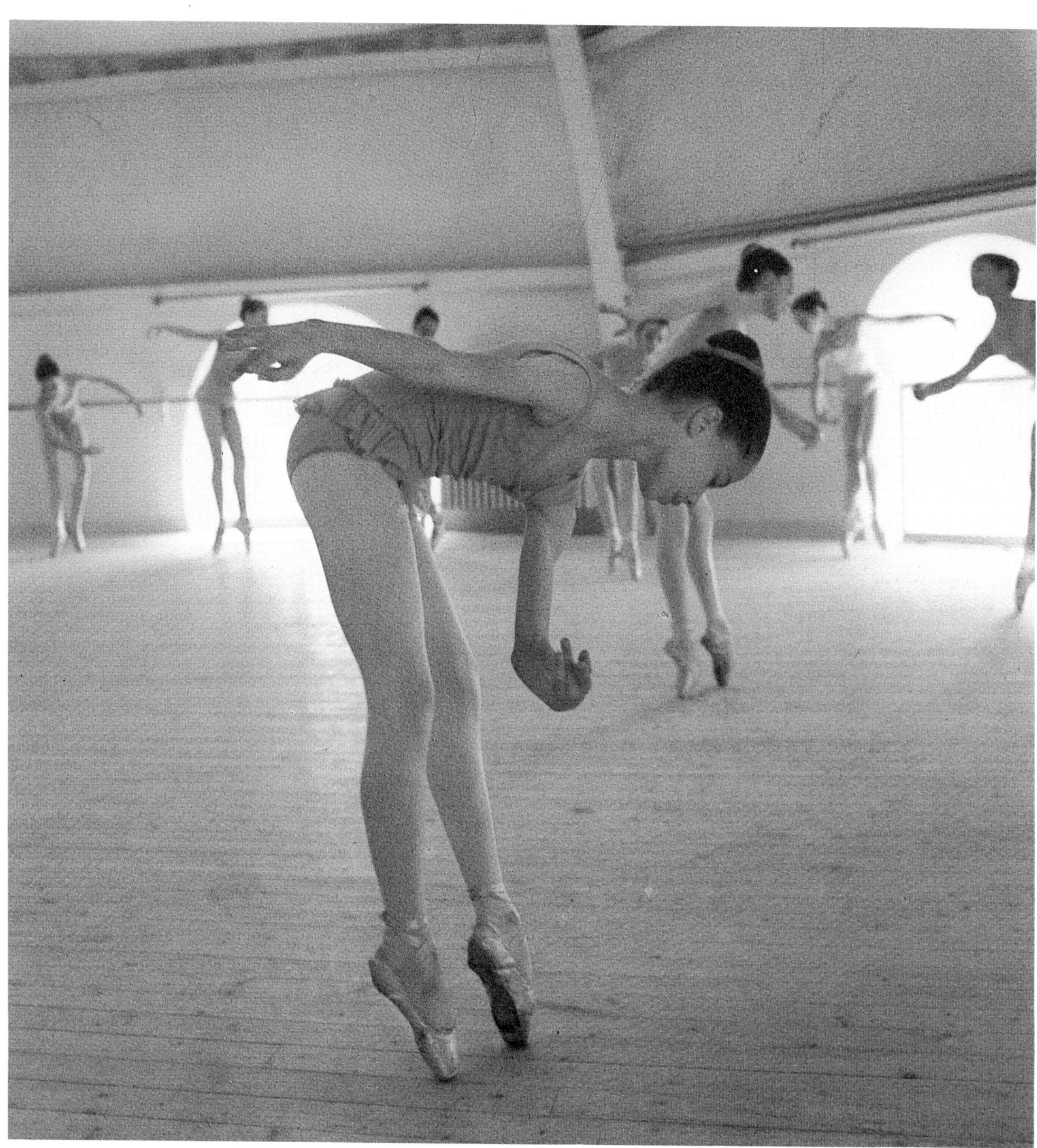

school of dance

3

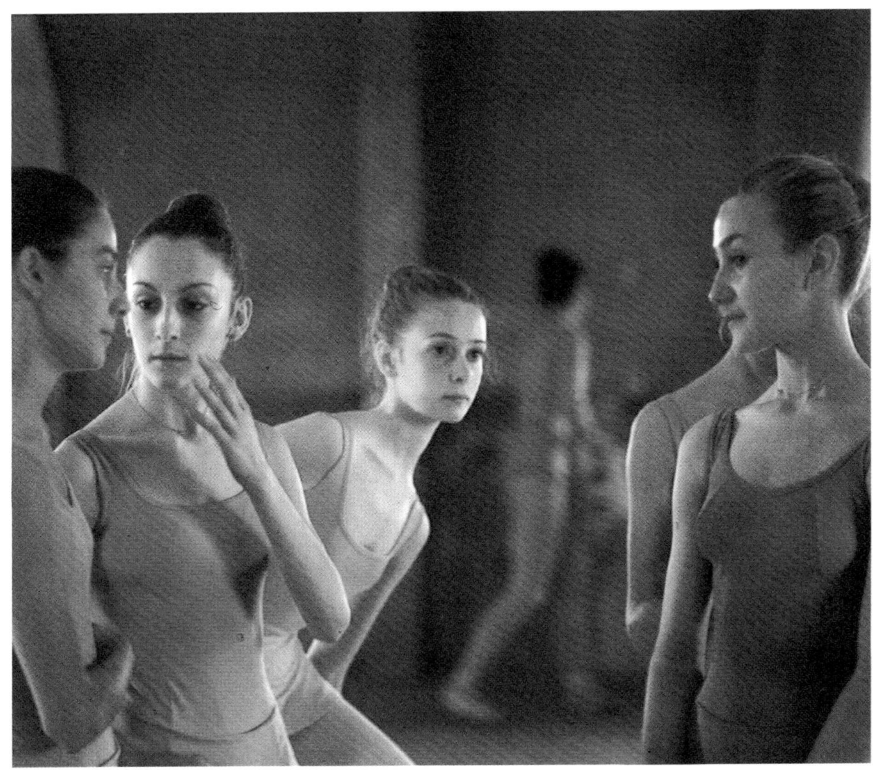

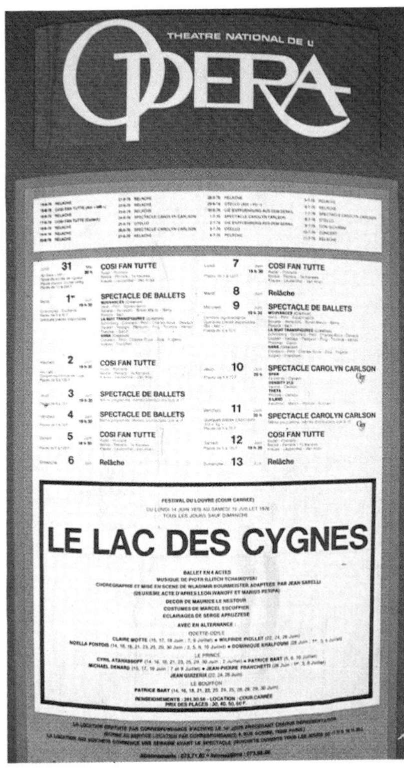

The Royal Academy of Dance was founded in 1661 during the reign of Louis XIV, and the School of Dance was founded in 1713. Since then the ballet has become an institution, and the company is one of the oldest in the world.

Today, after an entrance examination, children who enter the school are prepared for a career in dance, and it is from the school that the majority of the dancers in the "corps de ballet" have come.

Those students who are accepted into the "corps" are accepted "on probation" so that they can become familiar with dancing on stage. Competitions are held as openings in the higher levels become available.

The different levels are as follows : stagiaires (apprentice) - quadrille (particular group of dances) - coryphée (leader of a quadrille) - sujet (subject) - premier danseur (first dancer).

"Etoiles" (stars) are nominated by the governing body of the theatre, after having been proposed by the director of the dance.

At the Opéra School of Dance courses are given each morning by 5 male and 5 female teachers in each of 5 categories. Each teacher is available to teach all levels (Madame Chauviré is no exception).

The basic exercises are taught practically the same way by each teacher, although each brings his own particular style and sense of direction to his class.

The Paris Opéra

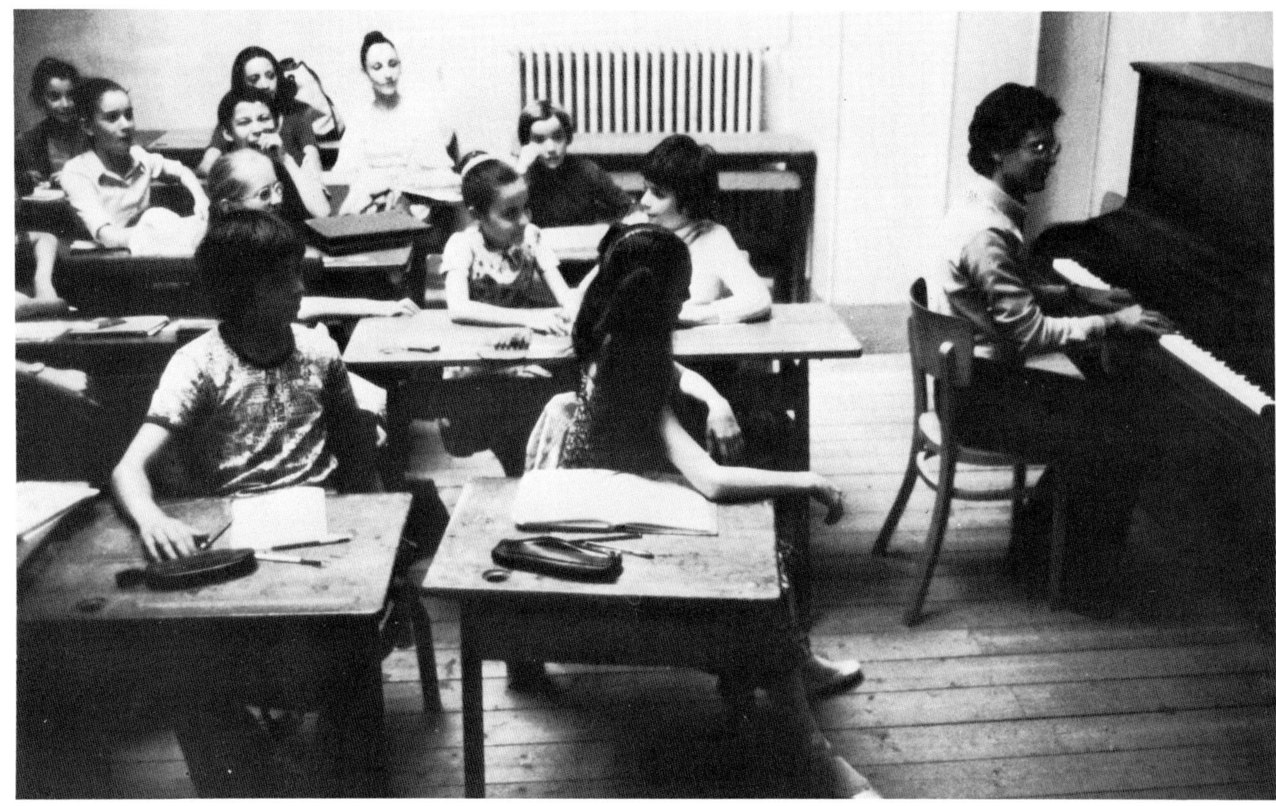

That is why the " corps de ballet ", born of the school itself, can readily adapt to the spirit and style of each choreographer invited by the Opéra.

Students at the school have a uniform for each class, and each child has the right to a new pair of slippers each month. At present there are about 100 students. Besides classes in dance, there are general courses of instruction as well.

The ballet of the Paris Opéra (second only to Moscow's Bolshoi) consists of 56 men, 74 women, and 13 " étoiles ", 6 of whom are men. The women retire at 40, the men at 45. There are no such restrictions for the " étoiles ".

The company of the Paris Opéra uses the talents of many famous choreographers and does not have an agreement with any one choreographer in particular.

The repertory consists of practically all the great traditional ballets as well as the many works of Maurice Béjart, George Balanchine, Jerome Robbins, Brian MacDonald, Carolyn Carlson, Roland Petit, etc...

The school of the Paris Opéra is under the direction of Madame Claude Bessy, a renowned ballerina and experienced leader.

school of dance

3

2

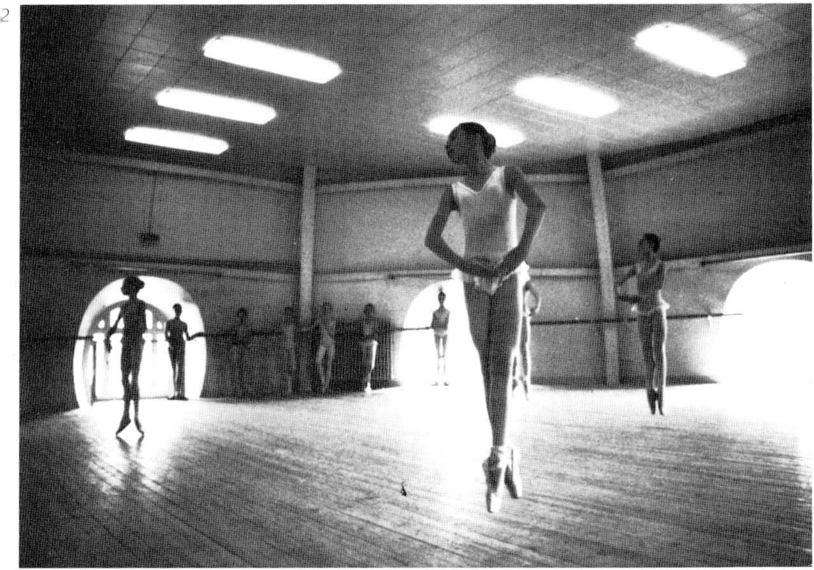

1 - A music class.

2-3 - A class
of Madame Gerodez.

4 - A class
of Madame Moreau.

3

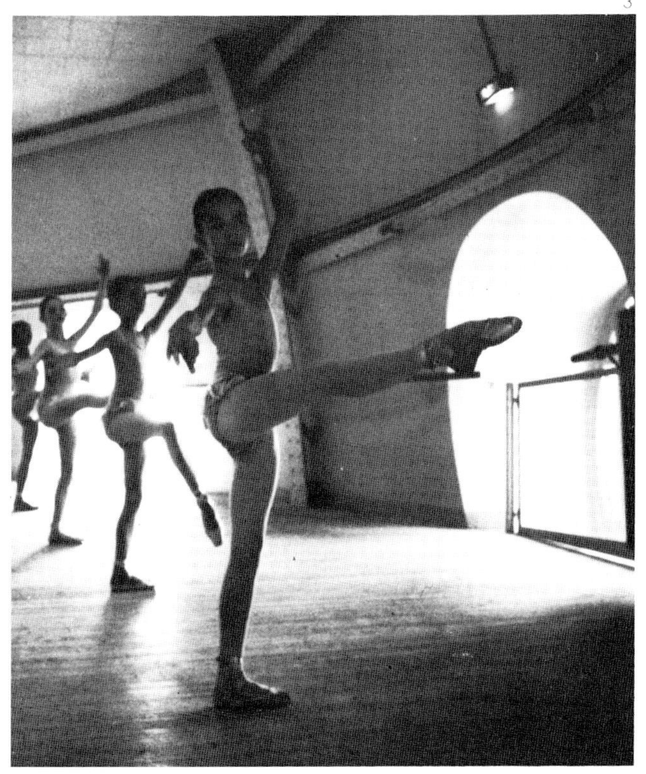

4

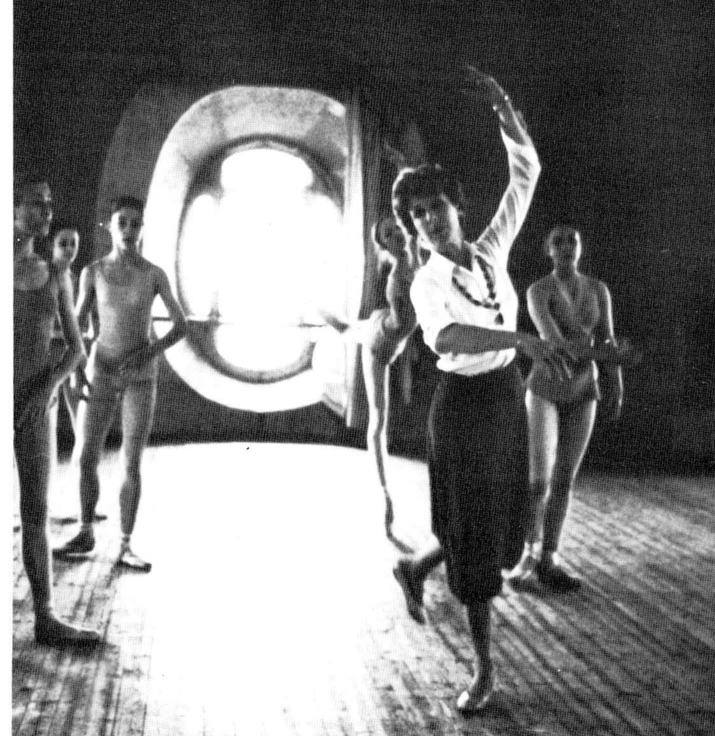

The most famous ballets

Giselle

Giselle, a ballet by Théophile Gautier and Vernoy de Saint-George, after a text by Heinrich Heine. Music by Adolphe Adam, choreography by Jean Coralli and Jules Perrot. Created for the Royal Academy of Paris, June 28, 1841. This is one of the most important ballets in the classical repertory. Since the ballerina must be both a fine dancer and a solid actress, this ballet is the supreme test of a young *étoile.*

In the shadow of a castle in the Rhine Valley live a young girl named Giselle and her mother. Two men are in love with Giselle-Hilarion, a gamekeeper, and Albrecht, a duke disguised as a peasant in order to win the favors of Giselle. Hilarion is very jealous of Albrecht and suspects that Albrecht is a noble.

The prince's hunting party arrives in the village, seeking shelter. In the party is the prince's daughter, Bathilde, to whom Albrecht is engaged to be married. Hilarion takes advantage of the prince's presence in the village to reveal the true identity of Albrecht. When Giselle, who is in love with Albrecht, hears of Albrecht's engagement to Bathilde and his different identity, she goes into a mad dance. She picks up Albrecht's sword—the evidence of his noble birth—and stabs herself. Giselle dies and joins the Wiles—ghosts of unmarried maidens who died because they danced too much before their wedding.

In the second act, Giselle rises from her tomb upon the command of Myrtha, the queen of the Wiles. Driven by guilt and crazed with despair, Albrecht follows her ghost in the hope of breaking the spell. In a trial, Myrtha condemns Hilarion to death and does so also to Albrecht. Hilarion is drowned but Giselle motions to Albrecht to seek safety by the cross on her grave. Angered by the defiance, Myrtha commands them both to dance an endless dance. Eventually, Albrecht falters and then falls from exhaustion. When the sun rises, he is found, overwhelmed with sorrow, lying on the tomb of his beloved.

Sleeping Beauty

This ballet is based on fairy tales by Charles Perrault. Music by Peter Tchaikovsky, choreography by Marius Petipa. First performed by the Russian Imperial Ballet in 1890 at St. Petersburg.

All the fairies of the kingdom, save one, have been invited to the castle for the baptism of Princess Aurora. On hand are the fairies of the Crystal Fountain, Enchanted Garden, Woodland Glades, Songbirds, and Golden Vine, as well as the Lilac Fairy. Each has brought as a gift a special promise of happiness and good fortune. Overlooked by the king and queen, however, is the evil fairy Carabosse. She enters the castle in a chariot drawn by large rats. Driven by revenge for not being invited, Carabosse promises that at age 16, Aurora will die by pricking her hand on a spindle.

The court is in an uproar. However, the Lilac Fairy tempers the wicked spell by transforming the prediction of death into one of sleep—a sleep that will last 100 years and will be broken only by the kiss of a handsome prince.

At the party given by the court to celebrate her 16th birthday, the young princess is given a gift of spindles by an old woman (Carabosse in disguise) and she pricks her finger and falls asleep amid the festivities. Soon after, everything stops. All members of the court, even the forest that surrounds the castle, fall into a deep slumber.

One hundred years later, the Lilac Fairy leads a handsome, charming prince through the sleeping forest to Aurora. Struck by her beauty, he wakens her with a magic kiss.

The ballet ends with their marriage, at which Aurora and the prince are entertained by dancers alluding to various other stories of Perrault (Puss'n Boots, etc.). It is one of the purest and most beautiful ballets in the repertory.

Costume by Varona for "Sleeping Beauty" at the Paris Opéra.

4

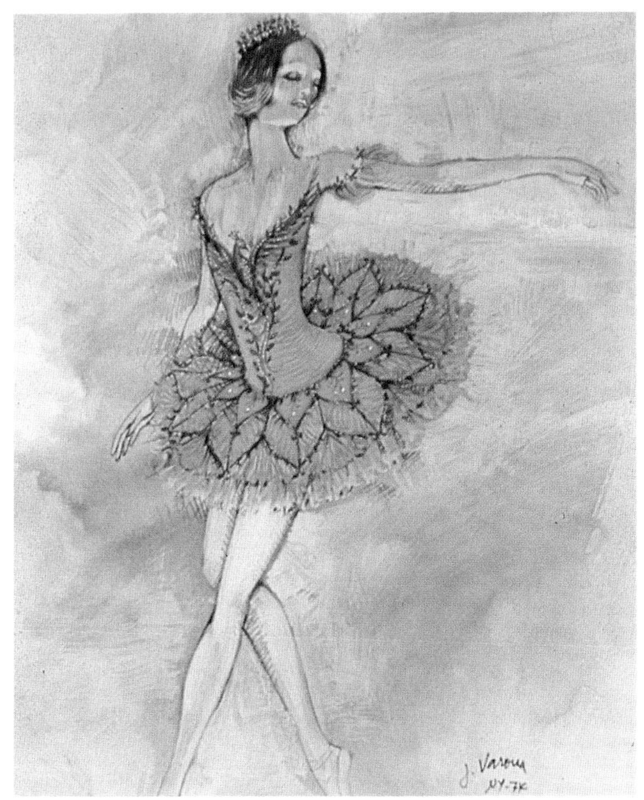

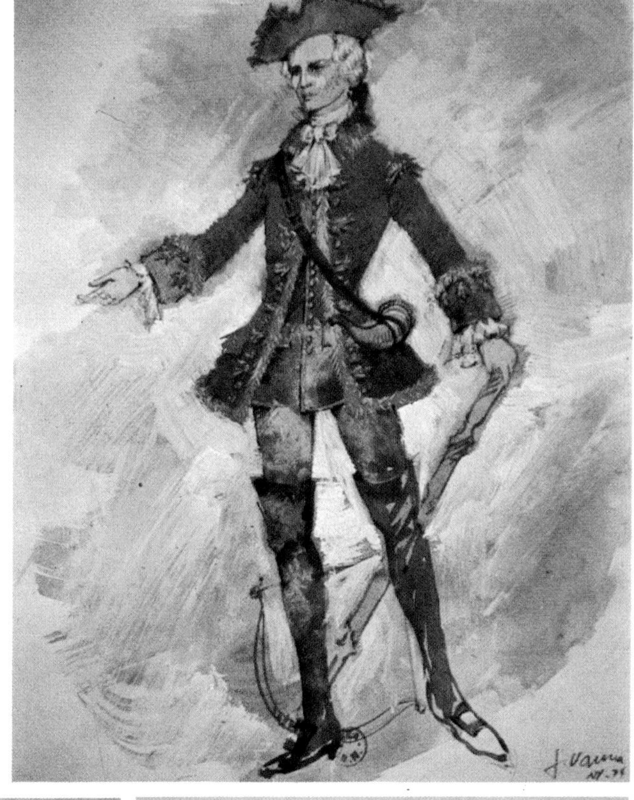

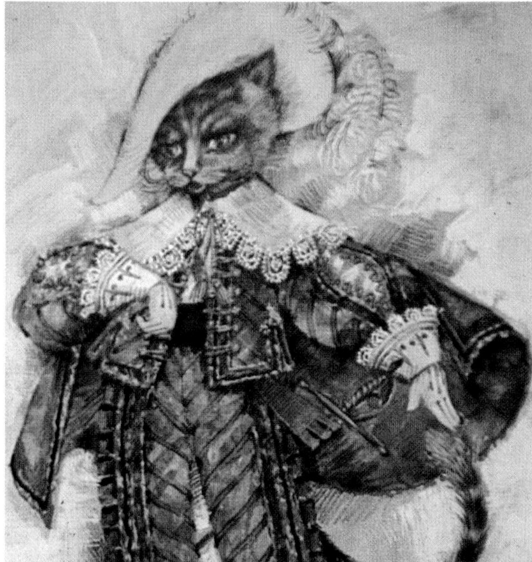

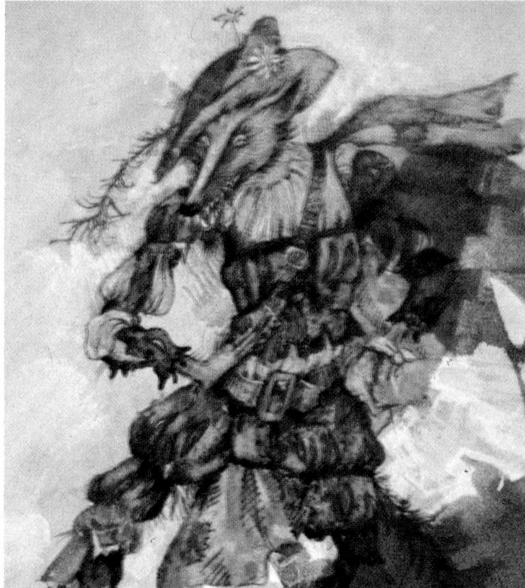

from left to right on the top:

Aurora and the prince.

from left to right on the bottom: Puss'n Boots and the Wolf (details).

The most famous ballets

Swan Lake

A frequently performed ballet based on the music of Peter Tchaikovsky. The version choreographed by Petipa and Ivanov was first presented by the Russian Imperial Ballet on January 17, 1895.

Prince Siegfried is celebrating his twenty-first birthday on the grounds of the palace: the following day he must choose his future bride. Night falls and the young man and his friends decide to go off hunting. In the woods, the prince sees a group of swans swimming on a lake. Just as he is about to draw his bow, he stops and the swans turn into beautiful young girls.

Odette, the swan queen, tells how she and the others are under a spell cast by a wicked magician. Only between midnight and dawn can they take on human shape, and only the love of a young man can free them from the curse. Siegfried falls deeply in love with the beautiful swan Odette. The magician appears and challenges Siegfried to prove his love for Odette. Siegfried swears his love and he then invites her to attend the ball to be given at the palace the next day.

At the ball there are many young girls invited by Siegfried's mother from whom she expects him to choose a bride. We see the young man refusing one prospective wife after another. Suddenly the wicked magician appears, disguised as a lord. Under his cloak he has hidden his daughter whom he has transformed into the exact likeness of Odette. He hopes to fool the prince into choosing her rather than the real princess, who has not yet appeared at the ball.

The prince does mistake the daughter for Odette and chooses her as his bride. As the magician and his daughter leave, Odette appears, revealing the trick. The choice has been made, however, and with death as their only escape from the evil magician, Siegfried and Odette flee through a storm and jump one after the other into the lake; they are re-united in death.

Coppelia

This ballet is derived from a tale of Hoffmann called "The Sand Merchant." The music is by Léo Delibes and choreography is by Arthur Saint-Léon. The ballet was first presented at the ancient home of the Paris Opéra on rue Lepeletier on May 25, 1870.

The youth of the village are intrigued by the immobile shape of a very beautiful young girl. She is seen sitting inside the window of the workshop of the elderly and illustrious toymaker Dr. Coppélius.

Taken by her beauty, young Franz keeps watch at the toymaker's house in the hope of attracting the attention of this mysterious girl. In order to get an even closer look, Swanilda, Franz's jealous fiancée, enters the workshop with her friends. She discovers that the pretty Coppélia is nothing more than an automaton, one of many the professor has created. Swanilda and her friends decide to have some fun with them.

Dr. Coppélius returns, and the girls flee —all except Swanilda, her curiousity aroused, who hides behind a curtain. At the same time, Franz appears, having climbed in through the window. Coppélius sees, in this unexpected visit, the chance to realize his greatest dream: to capture the essence of a human being and use it to bring one of his dolls to life.

Seizing the young man, he forces Franz to drink a vial of magic potion, and, after some wicked maneuvers, succeeds in passing the boy's spirit into one of his dolls. The doll (Swanilda in the doll's clothes) begins to move and proceeds to express all the beauty and joy of life in a dance. After a while, Swanilda wakes Franz and they flee together into the street. The doctor discovers that the doll indeed never did come to life. His dreams are shattered but the lord of the village gives him a bag of gold to compensate and there is merriment and dancing.

Costume by Varona for "Sleeping Beauty" at the Paris Opéra.

4

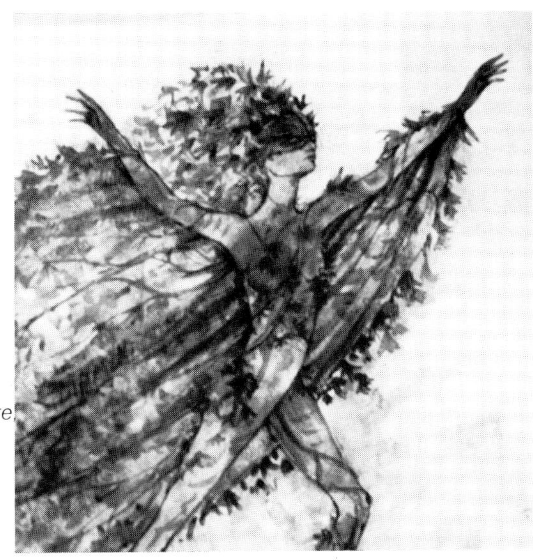

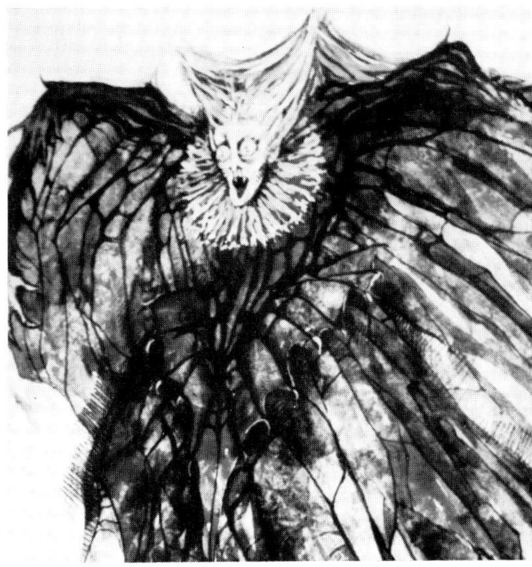

above,
from left to right:
the plant-like creature,
the fairy Carabosse.

below,
from left to right:
the king,
the queen.

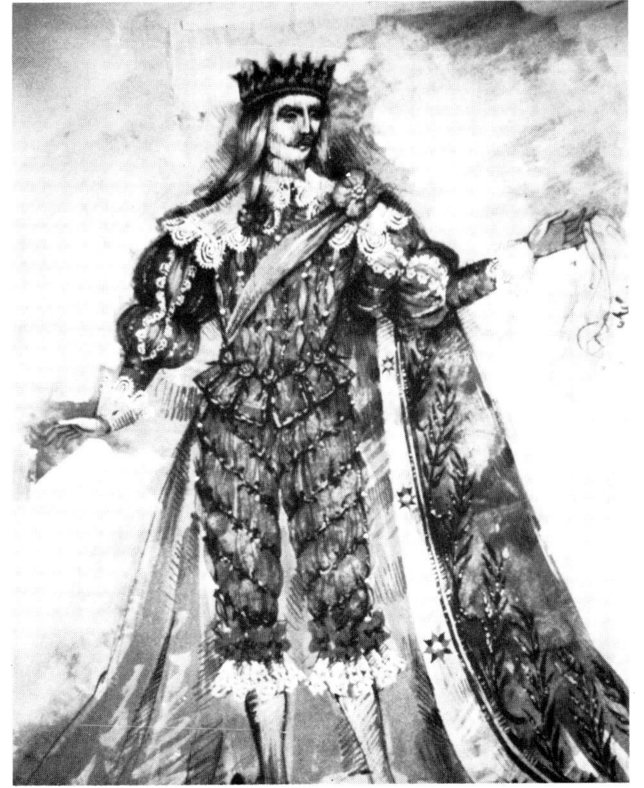

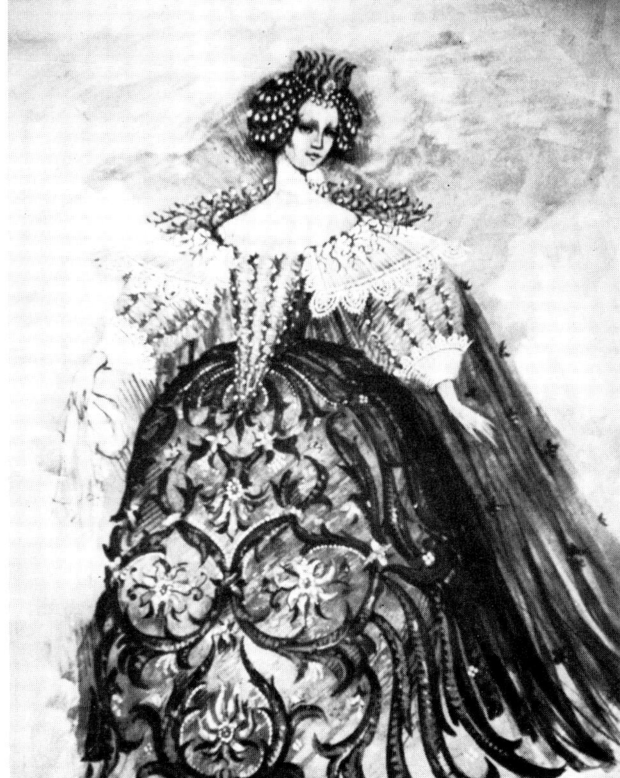

The great dancers

RUDOLF NUREYEV

A man of intense genius, Nureyev dominates the world of dance today. Born in a train on March 17, 1938, he began studying dance at the age of 11, in the Soviet Union. At age 17, he was accepted at the Leningrad Ballet School. Then he began dancing solo roles with the Kirov Ballet; it was during one of this company's tours in Paris that he elected to stay in Europe. Engaged by the Grand Ballet du Marquis de Cuevas for his brilliant troupe, Nureyev danced as the *étoile* in every ballet.

In 1962, he appeared for the first time with Margot Fonteyn in *Giselle.* The two dancers rapidly became a celebrated couple and since the 1960s, Nureyev's talents as both dancer and choreographer have been engaged by many of the world's great companies (including the Royal Ballet, the Vienna State Opera, and Béjart). Rudolf Nureyev is a dancer who possesses, among other abilities, extraordinary athletic qualities. He can leap higher than the majority of dancers and, in doing so, actually appears to be flying.

DAME MARGOT FONTEYN

Margot Fonteyn was born on May 18, 1919, in Surrey, England. She studied dance in Hong Kong and in London. She attended the Sadler's Wells Ballet School and made her debut in 1934 with the Vic-Wells Ballet. At this time, she began to take over the roles formerly danced by Alicia Markova, another outstanding ballerina.

Under the guidance of the famed choreographer Frederick Ashton, Fonteyn created leading roles in *The Sleeping Beauty, Horoscope, Daphnis and Chloë, Ondine, Firebird,* and *Petrouchka.* During the 1960s, she and her partner Rudolf Nureyev captured the attention of the entire world.

MAYA PLISETSKAYA

The most accomplished of the Russian dancers, Maya Plisetskaya is a star with the Bolshoi Ballet in Moscow, although her fame is far-reaching. Born in Moscow in 1925, she was schooled at the Bolshoi theatre. Her talents are great, for she is able to perfectly execute the most difficult steps. She has taken over the roles formerly danced by Galina Olanova and although she has been criticized as lacking lyricism, with movements perhaps a bit too violent, to many fans throughout the world she presents the image of the perfect ballerina.

ANTHONY DOWELL

Born February 16, 1943, Anthony Dowell is a principal dancer with the Royal Ballet. It is said of Dowell that he shows an amazing fluidity, coupled with a strong technique. His dramatic abilities are widely respected and he is very versatile. Although he suffered a cracked leg bone years ago, it has not prevented him from being a strong, exciting performer. His most notable performances to date have been in *The Dream, Romeo and Juliet, Card Game, Monotones.*

There are many other impressive dancers whose artistry shines throughout the world. For example, there are Yuri Soloviev, Mikhail Barishnikov, Valeri Panov, Merle Park, Natalia Makarova, Jacob Nielsen, Monica Mason, Edward Villella, Lynn Seymour, Antoinette Sibley, Carla Fracci, to mention but a few.

5

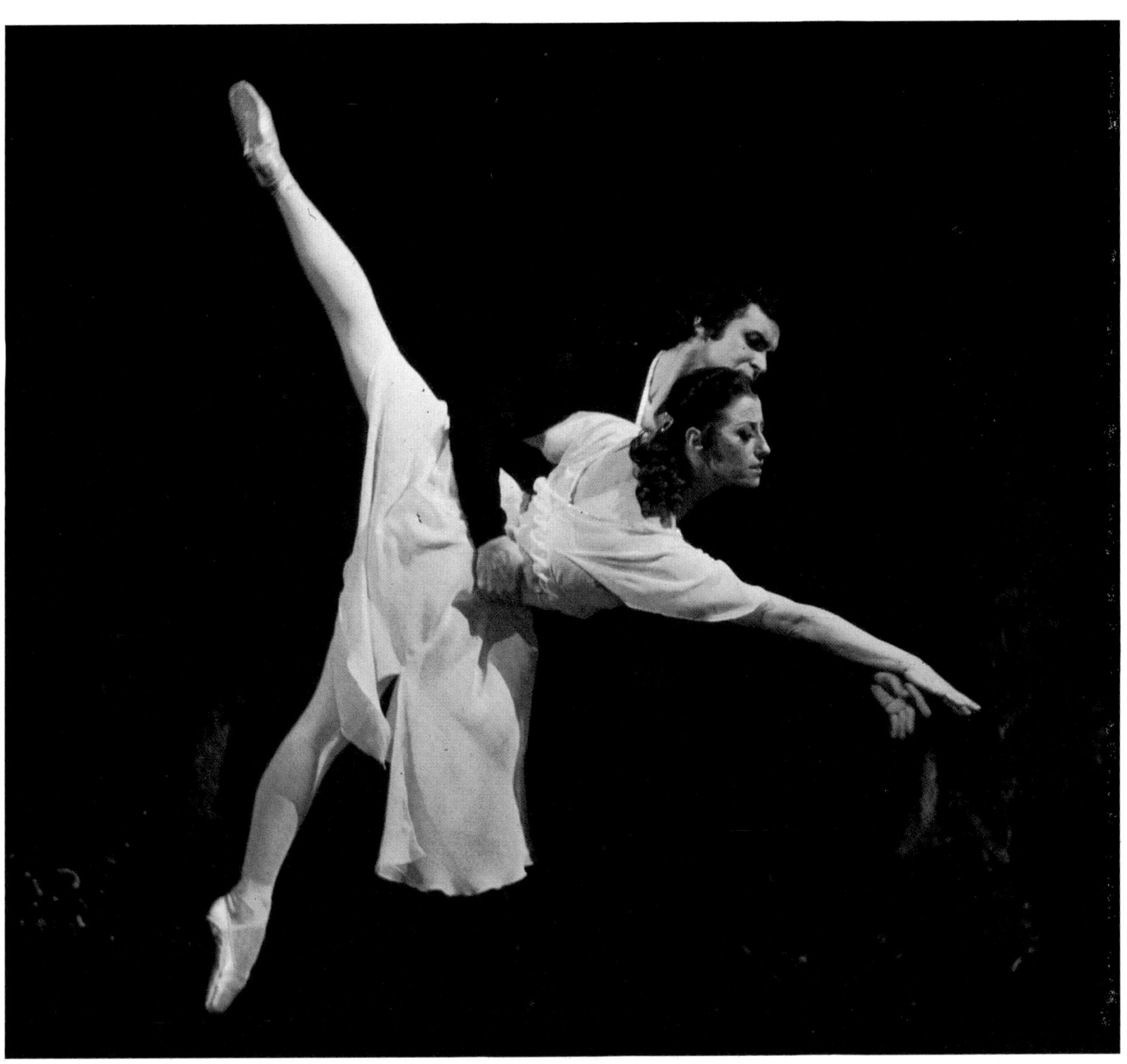

Maurice Béjart

Maurice Béjart is a master: one of the most innovative and talented creators alive today in the field of ballet. Thanks to him, the ballet has become more popular, particularly among the young. He brings to his ballets a sense of theatrical effect; his is a most individualistic choreography.

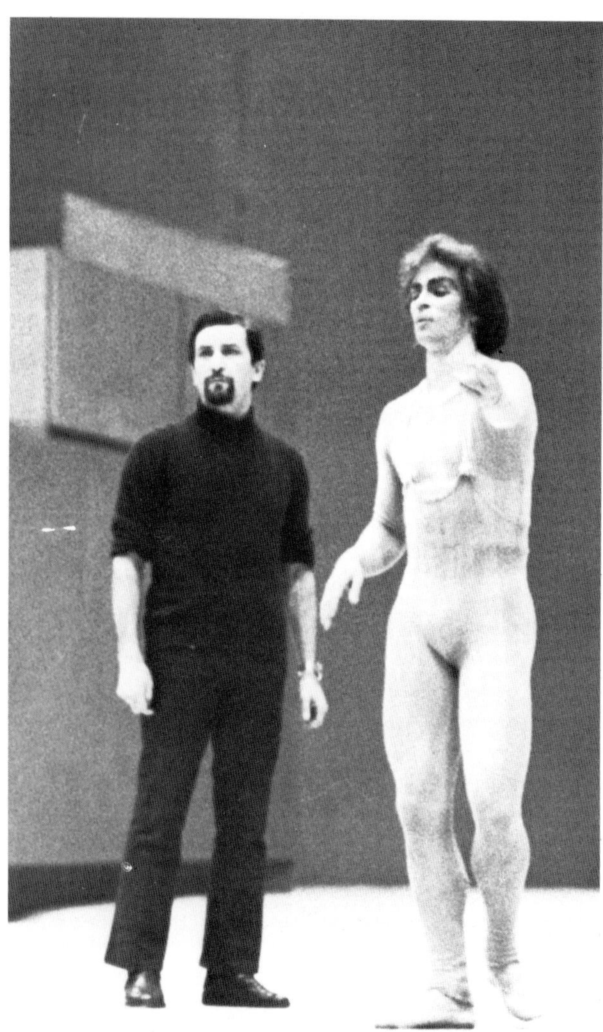

Maurice Béjart and Rudolf Nuryev

Originally from Marseilles, Maurice Béjart achieved status in 1955 with his *Symphony for One Man.* In the *Rite of Spring,* in 1959, Béjart found a perfect theme for his work. He presented movements that where simple but that stressed the basic eroticism of humanity. Later works were to continue to show this intensity often coupled with Indian classical dancing.

The home of his company, the Ballet of the Twentieth Century, is in Brussels, Belgium. It consists of 70 dancers, as well as the *étoiles* of other companies who appear as guest performers.

Principal Ballets

1955 *Symphonie pour un homme seul (Symphony for One Man).* Music by Pierre Schaeffer and Pierre Henry.
1957 *L'Etranger (The Stranger).* Music by Villa-Lobos.
1959 *Le Sacre du Printemps (Rite of Spring).* Music by Igor Stravinsky.
1960 *Boléro.* Music by Maurice Ravel.
1962 *Le Voyage (The Trip).* Music by Peter Henry.
1964 *9e Symphonie (Ninth Symphony).* Music by Beethoven.
1965 *Variations pour une porte et un soupir (Variations on an Entrance and a Sigh).* Music by Pierre Henry.
Erotica (A love Duet). Music by Tadeusz Baird.
1966 *Roméo et Juliette (Romeo and Juliet).* Music by Hector Berlioz.
1968 *Ni Fleurs ni Couronnes (Neither Flowers nor Crowns).* Based on choreographic themes of Marius Petipa and Peter Tchaikovsky.
Baudelaire. Music by Debussy, Wagner, and Pierre Henry.
Bhakti. Based on Hindu music themes.
1969 *Nomos Alpha.* Music by Iannis Xenakis.
1970 *L'Oiseau de feu (Firebird).* Music by Igor Stravinsky.
1971 *Nijinsky, Clown de Dieu (Nijinsky, Clown of God).* Music by Tchaikovsky and Pierre Henry.
1975 *Notre Faust (Our Faust).* Music by Johann Sebastian Bach and from Argentinian tangos.
1976 *Ce que l'amour me dit (What Love Tells Me).* Music by Gustav Mahler.

Roland Petit

6

Having trained at the Paris Opéra, Roland Petit is today the guiding spirit behind the ballet of the Marseilles Opéra. After the Paris Opéra, Petit's company is certainly the most important in France. Roland Petit entered the Paris Opéra School at 15 and left five years later. While there, and under the artistic patronage of Serge Lifar, he danced the lead in *L'Amour Sorcier (Bewitching Love).* In 1945, he directed the Ballet of the Champs-Elysées and became celebrated for his production of *Les Forains (The Strolling Players)* by Henri Sauquet. Another masterpiece, *Le Jeune Homme et la Mort (The Young Man and Death)* followed.

In 1948, he formed the Ballets de Paris de Roland Petit and a great number of ballets followed. It was at this time at that Janine Charrat began her brilliant career as a choreographer for the troupe, and talented people with whom he had already worked also joined him: Babilée, Algaroff, Tcherina, Etery, Pagava, and his future wife, Zizi Jeanmaire.

Today Petit continues to attract and involve talented dancers, further developing the artistry of each. In addition, he has staged ballets for other major companies, including the Royal Ballet and the Royal Danish Ballet.

Principal Ballets

1945 - *Les Forains (The Strolling Players).* Music by Henri Sauget. 1946 - *Le Jeune Homme et la Mort (The Young Man and Death).* Music by Johann Sebastian Bach. 1948 - *Les Demoiselles de la Nuit (The Young Ladies of Midnight).* Music by Jean Francaix. 1949 - *Carmen.* Music by Georges Bizet. *L'Oeuf à la Coque (The Soft-Boiled Egg).* 1950 - *La Croqueuse de Diamants (The Diamond Cruncher).* Music by Jean-Michel Damase, lyrics by Ramond Queneau. 1952 - *Deuil en 24 Heures (In Mourning for 24 Hours).* 1953 - *Le Loup (The Wolf).* Music by Henri Dutilleau. 1961 - *Cyrano de Bergerac.* Music by Marius Constant. 1962 - *Maldoror.* 1965 - *Notre-Dame de Paris.* 1966 - *L'Eloge de la Folie (An Elogy on Madness).* 1967 - *Paradise Lost.* Music by Marius Constant. 1968 - *Turangalila. 1972 - Pink Floyd Ballet, Allumez les Etoiles (Light Up the Stars).* 1974 - *Les Intermittences du Cœur.* Based on the work of Marcel Proust. 1975 - *La Symphonie Fantastique.* Music by Hector Berlioz. *Coppélia.* Music by Léo Delibes. 1976 - *Nana.*

Loïja Araujo and Denis Ganio in "Coppelia". Choreorgraphy by Roland Petit for the Ballets of Marseille.

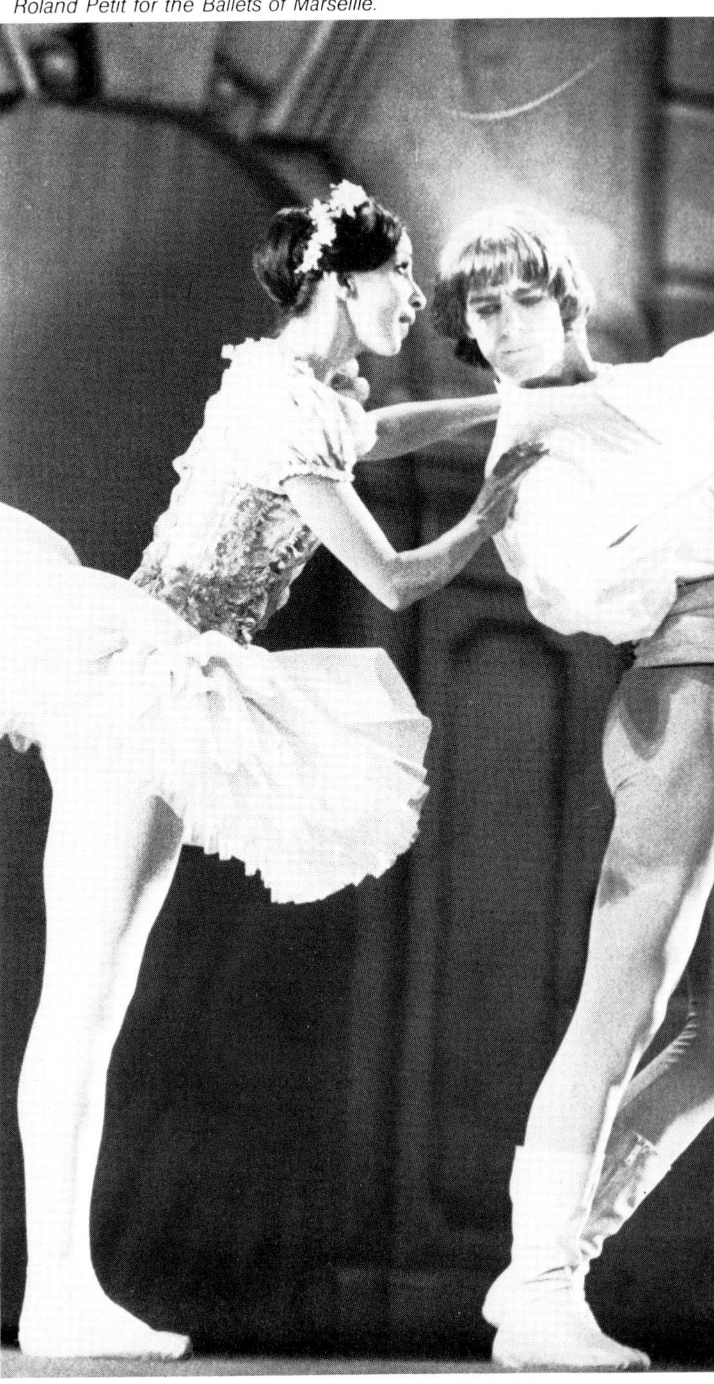

Great American

GEORGE BALANCHINE

George Balanchine, born on January 9, 1904 in Leningrad, is the personality who dominates the world of dance today. Trained at the Imperial School of Ballet, he was first brought to the world's attention by Diaghilev, one of the men responsible for popularizing the Russian ballet abroad.

Since that time, Balanchine has become leader of the New York City Ballet; he is the author of more than 100 ballets that are performed throughout the world. Among the most notable of his works are *The Nutcracker* and *Don Quixote.*

Balanchine is a varied artist. He has worked with modern composers such as Schoenberg, Ives, and Stravinsky. He has also contributed to other arts; for example, he choreographed the dance sequences for the movie *Slaughter on Tenth Avenue* and the Broadway production, *On Your Toes.* In each of his productions, Balanchine brings out a strong sense of musicality and an intense concern with linear purity.

MARTHA GRAHAM AND HER PUPILS

Born on May 11, 1893, Martha Graham is probably the most influential American on the art of dance. She has been an inspiration for her pupils—most notably Merce Cunningham and Paul Taylor. As an innovator creating and refining the techniques of modern dance, Graham has moved in the eyes of the public from controversial to highly established. She has been working for over 50 years, either as a dancer, a choreographer, or a teacher, and she has created over 150 works, taken mostly from history, literature, and mythology.

Merce Cunningham

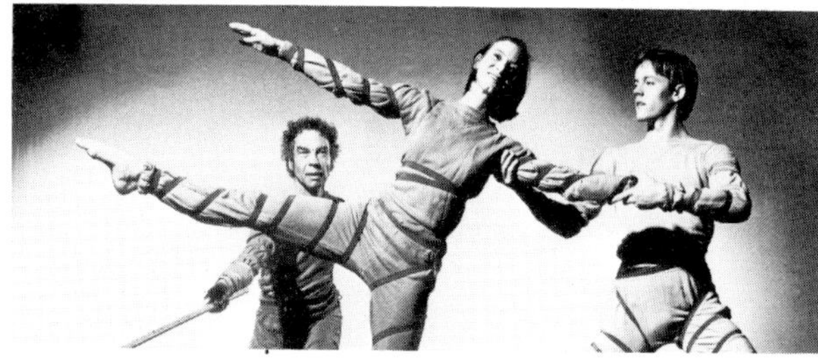

Merce Cunningham and Paul Taylor danced formerly with Martha Graham's company and their styles, although different, reflect aspects of Graham's influence. Cunningham's works have been said to be described as serenely abstract, while Taylor's are unrestrained and impassioned. Whereas Cunningham works into his ballets the element of chance and invention, Taylor uses classic and simplified classical steps. Cunningham is known for such works as *Un Jour ou Deux (One Day or Two);* Taylor's *Orb* has received critical acclaim.

JEROME ROBBINS

Jerome Robbins is the most celebrated of American-born choreographers. He is the originator of a style that uses everyday happenings as its source. Robbins has had a varied career; he has danced all types of ballets, from classical, to modern, to Oriental. He is very well known for the choreography he did for the film *West Side Story,* but the productions he did with the New York City Ballet from 1949 through 1963 have also received praise. Two productions of his, *Afternoon of a Faun* and *Dances at a Gatherings,* particularly are said to reflect Robbin's subtle sense of humor.

Louis Falco.

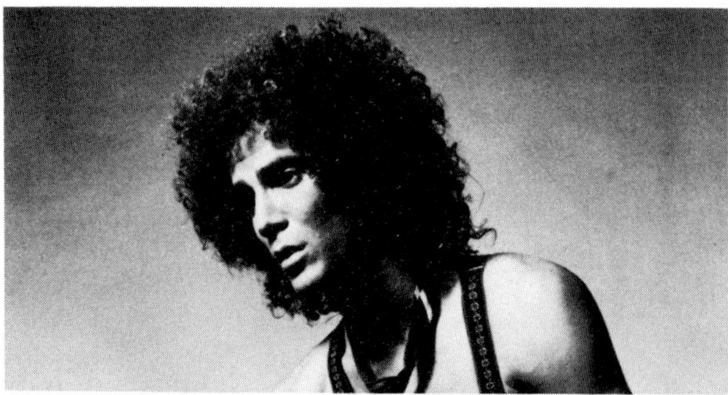

ALVIN AILEY

Alvin Ailey is a black American born in Texas. Today he is head of the Alvin Ailey City Center Dance Theatre, one of America's most important dance companies.

Ailey's contributions to dance are unique. He has brought to the stage the aspects of American Negro culture often ignored by the rest of society. His company includes some great Negro dancers, especially Judith Jamison and William Louther. One of Ailey's most highly acclaimed pieces is his *Revelations,* set to the music of Negro spirituals.

choreographers

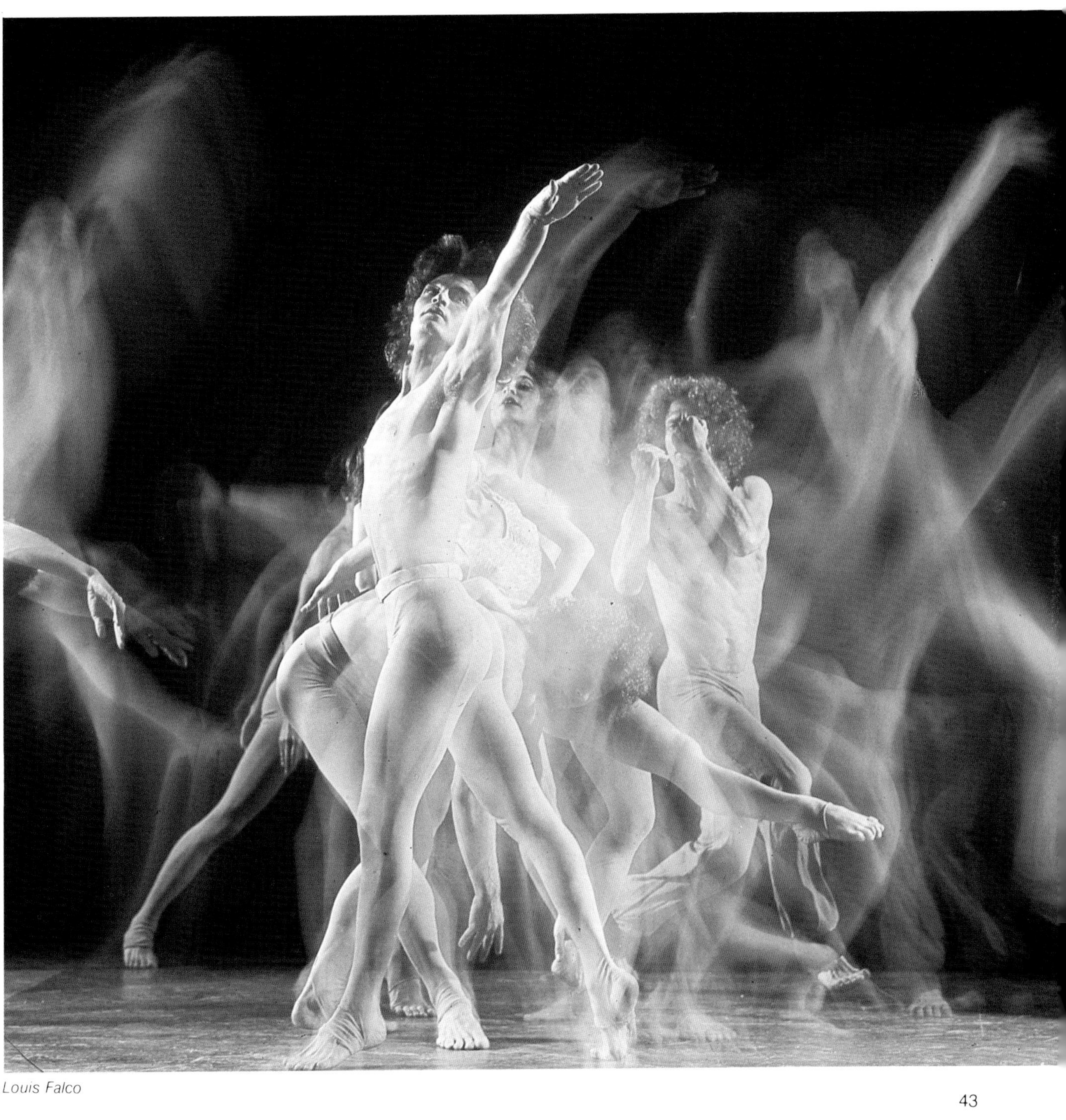

Louis Falco

Backstage

The ballet employs many people who are rarely seen.

A dancer's legs are precious and fragile. They are as important to him as an instrument is to a musician. At the slightest pain the dancer rushes to a "masseur" to have the dislocations and sprains repaired so that he can dance again... quickly!

Dance slippers are very important, and their fit must be exact. The ribbons, which can be tied in many different ways, are virtually destroyed after each performance. The "étoiles" often give them to admirers. The majority of slippers used to be made in Italy, but today they come from all over. They cost about 12 dollars or 6 pounds.
Speciality shops sell cotton and wool stockings for practice, and silk stockings for performances.
The "tutus", skirts of ruffled muslin, are either made in the theatres or by special costume houses.
There exist for the ballet, as for the theatre, specialists who create costumes and design sets.

Special rehearsals are given for the benefit of dance photographers. Besides working for the press, these photographers sell their prints to the artists or to the public as posters.
Photographing the dance is difficult. Imagine the skill it takes to capture the subtlest movement, or the end of a leap.

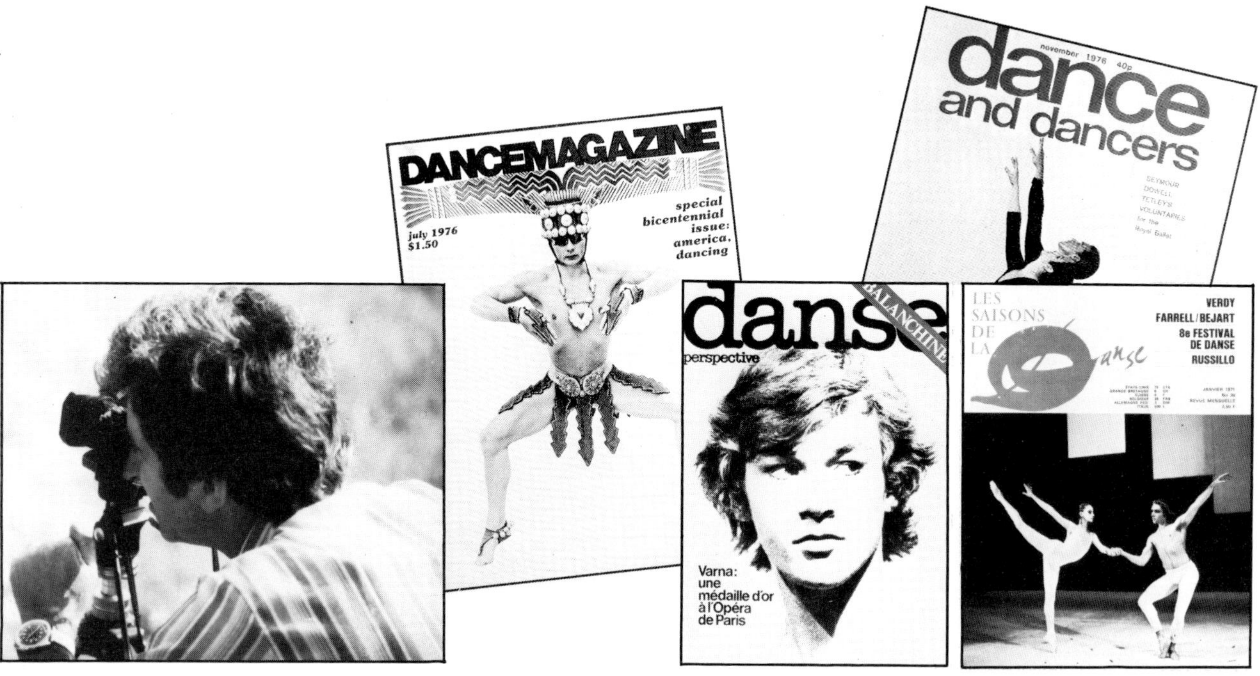

There are also magazines that specialize in choreography. In France, there are two : *Les Saisons de la Danse* and *Danse Perspective.* In the United States, the major magazine for people interested in dance is *Dance Magazine.* Dance journalists attend all performances and they are always on the lookout for new talent.

Schools

8

United States

You will find a more extensive listing of dance schools in the back issues of *Dance Magazine*. In addition, many undergraduate colleges throughout the country offer programs in dance and many of these programs lead to a bachelor of fine arts degree. The following listing is a brief one, indicating a few schools located in various parts of the country.

LOS ANGELES BALLET - 11843 W. Olympic Blvd. Los Angeles, California 90064.
SAN FRANCISCO BALLET SCHOOL - 378 18th Avenue, San Francisco, California 94121.
DENVER BALLET ACADEMY - No 2 Broadway, Denver, Colorado 80203.
HARTFORD BALLET COMPANY - 308 Farmington Avenue, Hartford, Connecticut 06105.
BOSTON CONSERVATORY OF MUSIC - 8 The Fenway, Boston, Massachusetts 02215.
INTERLOCHEN ARTS ACADEMY - Interlochen, Michigan 49643.
NEW JERSEY SCHOOL OF BALLET - 300 Main Street, Orange, New Jersey 07050.
ALVIN AILEY AMERICAN DANCE CENTER - 229 East 59th Street, New York, New York 10023.
HARKNESS SCHOOL OF BALLET - 4 East 75th Street New York, New York 10021.
NEW YORK ACADEMY OF BALLET AND DANCE ARTS - 667 Madison Avenue at 61 Street, New York, New York 10021.
PRATT INSTITUTE - 215 Ryerson Street, Brooklyn, New York 11201.
MARTHA GRAHAM SCHOOL OF CONTEMPORARY DANCE - 316 East 63rd Street, New York, New York 10021.
OKLAHOMA CITY METROPOLITAN BALLET SCHOOL - 2501 N. Blackwelder, Oklahoma City, Oklahoma 73106.
DALLAS BALLET ACADEMY - 3601 Rawlins, Dallas, Texas 75291.

Great-Britain

BALLET FOR ALL - Alexander Grant, director. Royal Opera House, Covent Gdn, London WC2E 7QA.
BALLET RAMBERT - Dame Marie Rambert DBE, John Chesworth, directors Prudence Skene, administrator; Adam Gatehouse, mus. dir. 94 Chiswick High Rd, London W4 ISH.
BALLETS MINERVA - Edward Gaillard, administr. Wembley Institute, London Road, Wembley HA9 7EX.
CONTEMPORARY DANCE TRUST LTD - Robert Cohan, Robin Howard, Jack Norton dirs. 17 Dukes Road, London WC1H 9AB.
CONTEMPORARY OPERA CO. - Tony Dinner, artistic dir.; Donal Rappoport, mus. dir. 79 Stanhope Av., London N3 3LY.
DANCE FOR EVERYONE - Naomi and David Hadda. 22 Mapesbury road, London W1H 3FA.
DANCE THEATRE COMMUNE - Ernest and Ailsa Berk, dirs. 52 Dorset St., London NW2 4JD.
INTERNATIONAL BALLET CARAVAN-ALEXANDER ROY BALLET THEATRE - Alexander Roy, artistic dir. 69 Eton Av., London NW3 3EU.
LONDON CONTEMPORARY DANCE THEATRE - Robert Cohan, artistic dir.; Janet Eager, administr. The Place, 17 Dukes road, London WC1H 9AB.
LONDON FESTIVAL BALLET TRUST LTD - Beryl Grey CBE, artistic dir.; Terence, Kern, prin cond. 48 Welbeck street, London W1M 7HE.
NEW LONDON BALLET - David Martin, administr. dir.; André Presser, mus. dir. 406 Harrow Road, London W9 2HU.
NORTHERN DANCE THEATRE - Freda Steel, administr. 11 Zion Cres, Hulme Walk, Manchester M15 EBY.
ROYAL BALLET - Kenneth MacMillan, dir.; Ashley Lawrence, mus. dir. Royal Opera House, Covent Gdn, London WC2E 7QA.
SEPHIROTH - Nikki Cole, dir. Dance Center, 12 Floral St., London WC2E 9DH.

France

ACADEMIE INTERNATIONALE DE DANSE (International Dance Academy) - Under the direction of Nicole Chirpaz.
ACADEMIE D'ART CHOREGRAPHIQUE RAYMOND FRANQUETTI - (Raymond Franquetti Academy of Choreographic Art) Professor, R. Franquetti, teacher at the Paris Opéra, 4 bis Cité Véron, 75018 Paris.
TESSA BEAUMONT - Classical dance for children, amateurs, professionals. Modern dance, tap, mime, exercise. 20, rue Guersant, 75017 Paris.
SOLANGE GOLOVINE - ACADEMIE DE DANSE (Dance Academy) - Sister of the celebrated dancer Serge Golovine, who also teaches at the Academy. 6, avenue George V, 75008 Paris.
CENTRE DE DANSE INTERNATIONAL (International Dance Center) - Rosella Hightower. Résidence Le Gallia, 06400 Cannes.
CENTRE DE DANSE DE PARIS (Dance Center of Paris) - Paul and Yvonne Goubé. Professors, Serge Peretti, of Paris Opéra, Rita Thalia, of the Paris Opĕra, Yvonne Meyer, Jeanine Monin. Salle Pleyel, 252 faubourg Saint-Honoré, 75008 Paris.

DANCE VOCABULARY

ADAGE
A combination of slow movements wherin the dancer seeks the purity of bodily lines, balance, and lyrical expression.

ATTERRISSAGE
Instant when, after a leap, a dancer makes contact with the floor.

BALLON
Elasticity at the end and the beginning of leaps.

BATTERIE
Term encompassing all the various "entrechats", any movement in which the legs cross while in the air.

CAMBRÉ
Movement for achieving greater suppleness during which the upper body bends forward, to the sides, and to the back.

CHOREOGRAPHY
Group of steps and gestures which make up a ballet.

CODA
The end of a ballet or the conclusion of a "pas de deux".

CHASSÉ
By sliding, one foot takes the place of the other.

DÉBOULÉS
A series of movements, generally excuted on the diagonal or around the circumference of the stage, during which the dancer rapidly turns.

DESCENDRE
To move towards the public. "Remonter" is the exact opposite : to go towards the back of the stage.

ÉTOILE
An artist with a world reputation, one who is considered to have perfected the dance.

FOUETTÉS
Series of rapid turns in place, with one leg constantly giving an outward thrust or kick.